T0312341

The
Natural
Facelift

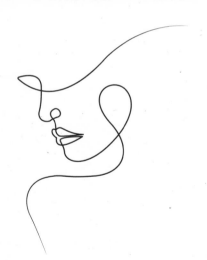

The Natural Facelift

Sculpt your face at home
in just 5 minutes a day

Sophie Perry

HarperCollins*Publishers*

HarperCollins*Publishers*
1 London Bridge Street
London SE1 9GF

www.harpercollins.co.uk

HarperCollins*Publishers*
Macken House, 39/40 Mayor Street Upper
Dublin 1, D01 C9W8, Ireland

First published by HarperCollinsPublishers 2024

3 5 7 9 10 8 6 4 2

A catalogue record of this book is available from the British Library

ISBN 978-0-00-865420-7

Printed and bound in the UK using 100% renewable
electricity at CPI Group (UK) Ltd

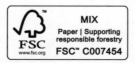

In honour of my mother – thank you for absolutely everything.

Contents

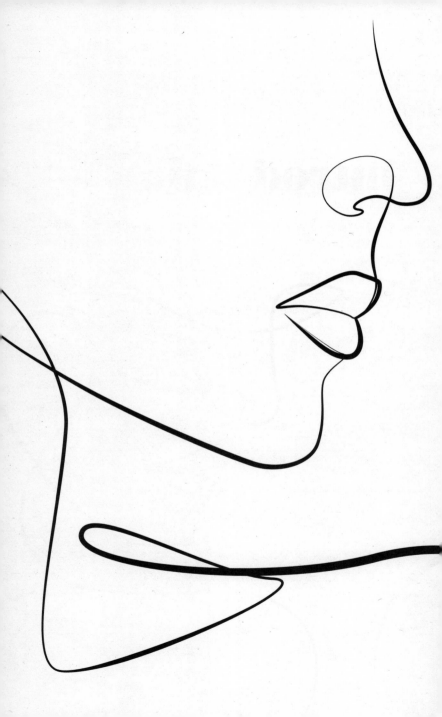

Introduction

Thank you for picking up this book, and for trusting me to act as your guide into the world of facial practices.

The beauty industry has a way of teaching us to look in the mirror and find 'flaws', rather than embrace our unique beauty. It's supposed to boost our confidence, yet it seems to thrive on our insecurities: expression lines that need erasing, lips that should be fuller, skin that must look flawless and clear ... But isn't ageing a privilege? A blessing? Something to welcome, enjoy and take pride in?

After many years of finding my way in this industry, my mission now is to be a voice that teaches everyone to love their uniqueness – not an easy task, I know! But I intend to change the way we talk about 'anti-ageing' and 'age prevention', which I've always seen as such negative terms. I believe we should all accept and enhance the features we are blessed with, strengthen our natural contours and celebrate our individuality.

I have written this book as an antidote to the fear that has taken root in many conversations about ageing, offering ways to promote your natural glow and vibrancy without damaging your face or your confidence in the process. Yes, I do offer practices that will help to reduce the signs of ageing, but with an emphasis that this comes first and foremost from a love for your skin and not from a place of fear. The practices certainly will not erase every line or wrinkle, but hopefully, after reading this book, you will feel like you wouldn't want that anyway. Because those lines are testament to a life well lived. And there is so much to love in our faces as they age and mature, while at the same time working to boost the health of our skin and enhance our favourite features.

What is 'The Natural Facelift'?

Quite simply, it is my personal guide to boost the skin you're in, naturally.

It will help you to understand how your skin works and the important structures that lie beneath what you see in the mirror. A knowledge of the anatomy of your facial muscles and the different layers of skin will arm you with what you need to work *with* your face, rather than *against* it. Even as a professional, I was taught about the skin itself, but not so much about the scaffolding and frame that help to hold it in place: namely, the muscles. When you work a bit deeper into your face, not just superficially, your skin will reap the benefits, as the firmer and healthier the facial muscles become, so too does the skin. Therefore, what better place to start?

In these pages, I offer many simple, natural practices you can do yourself at home to help improve your skin's health and function – whatever your skin type – including massage and facial exercises. These two techniques together help to boost the function of your body's natural processes and responses, so that you feel and look your best. They are all things you can do with no equipment (as I always say, your hands are your best tools), although I have also included a list of tools you might consider trying if you're interested (see p. 43).

* **Massage** We all know that body massage can do wonders for releasing built-up tension in the body, flushing blood through the muscles and releasing blockages from strain and overuse. But although we're aware of how this works for the body, we often forget that the same principles can be applied to the face. Facial massage is incredibly beneficial for restoring mobility to facial muscles which, because of modern life, are not being exercised enough. Think, for example, of how many hours a day you might sit frowning at a computer screen, your phone or TV – facial muscles can easily stiffen, causing potential blockages (say, in the lymphatic system), discomfort and headaches and entrenched fine lines. Massage can be wonderful for keeping blood flowing, draining the lymphatic system and enhancing features by reducing puffiness.

* **Facial exercises** Similarly, most of us understand how workouts or yoga benefit the body, particularly those of us who do exercises focused on a specific muscle group – when targeting one area, you can often see results in tone or bulk pretty quickly. The same applies to the face, yet most workouts stop below the neck. In day-to-day living, many facial muscles do not get the right sort of exercise, which can result in them becoming looser,

so that the skin appears less firm. The practices you will find in this book target the right muscles to help lift and tone some, while relaxing others.

These techniques focus on the structure of the face. They dig deep, isolating individual muscle groups to manipulate, energise, destress, redefine and strengthen, while targeting the connective tissues to improve skin function and health. They are natural treatments that provide incredible confidence-boosting results for all skin types and complexions, improving the efficiency of natural bodily functions, enhancing uniqueness and benefiting health and wellness in so many ways. And the best part? It is all from the comfort of your own home.

The benefits

I'm beyond passionate about the practices in the book, and these are just some of the results you might expect to see or feel:

* **A glowing, vibrant, healthy-looking complexion**
  The practices here can be hugely beneficial in supporting the circulatory system, to help boost in healthy oxygen and nutrients, providing your skin with all the goodness it needs to survive and flourish – making it brighter in the process.
* **More plump, youthful skin with smoothed-out wrinkles** The lymphatic system is supported by

promoting the drainage of excess fluid, which
detoxifies and then renews the skin. The system itself
doesn't have a pump, so facial massage really gives it
a helping hand.

* **More defined features and improved muscle tone**
Puffiness is reduced when the lymphatic system
gets going, but the facial muscles are also worked,
so that they become firmer (in the same way that
bicep curls tone your arms). The facial exercises will
particularly help to give you a more defined jawline
and cheekbones, bringing out the natural contours of
your face, as well as reducing the appearance of circles
under the eyes.

* **Fewer breakouts** Through detoxifying the skin and
stimulating blood flow, you will be able to reduce the
appearance of acne and even help to prevent it.

* **Releasing tension and reducing stress** This point often
surprises people, as many do not realise how much
stress we hold in our facial muscles. We know how it
feels to hold tension throughout the body – upper-
back pain from holding heavy bags, for example, or
lower-back and hip pain from lifting children – but
what about the muscles of the face? There is often a
lot of tension that comes from day-to-day life, whether
you work at a computer screen all day and your eyes
feel the strain or you live or work in a high-stress
environment and find yourself clenching your jaw.
Perhaps you didn't even realise until you read this –
that's right, loosen that jaw … I see you!

Our skin can fall victim to stress just as much as the rest of the body. Stress accelerates ageing, impacting the skin's strength and elasticity, as well as increasing the inflammatory response in those who suffer with conditions like eczema or acne. But the practices in this book can release tension and stress, relax the nervous system and reduce anxiety – all of which has a positive effect on your skin.

About me

I have over 14 years' experience in this industry – although, I'll be honest, the term 'the beauty industry' will never sit well with me as it can sound so superficial, and we know it can offer so much more than that. I have always had a bit of a love-hate relationship with it, but now that I've found what works for me, it only feels natural to share that with others.

I started my career as an aesthetic practitioner, performing many treatments (things like laser hair removal, facial rejuvenation in the form of microneedling, chemical peels, facial massage and more lasers) and building a wonderful client base – clients who became friends. We used non-invasive body treatments to tone, tighten and firm; specialised deep-tissue massages to reduce pain such as sciatica; and pregnancy massage. All these treatments had one thing in common: to help make someone *feel* their best; and working in this industry, there's no better feeling than seeing your client beam from ear to ear with happiness over the results of what you helped them achieve. That's job satisfaction right there, and I'm sure my fellow practitioners can agree.

But it's not just about the practical side of treatments; building a rapport with clients means building connections, forming relationships and trust. The treatment room is a safe haven in which to unwind and destress, offload daily struggles and feel lighter mentally. I loved this part of my work and still do, to this day. But it wasn't until I started teaching others in my field of work, watching them learn, develop new skills, grow and gain the same satisfaction, that I realised my true passion lay not just in the industry itself, but also in teaching others how to get the most out of it.

The journey from treating to education was a real learning curve for me. I progressed and moved into assisting in the medical field, gaining an awareness and understanding of more invasive treatments. All of which provided clients with a confidence boost that was incredible to witness and be a part of. However, it was also at this time in my career that I began to question the industry and my place within it.

I found myself in rooms with medical professionals who were suggesting intense treatments for areas of the face the client hadn't even thought about and certainly hadn't 'realised' were cause for 'concern' visually. How was that beneficial? Didn't it contradict what the industry stood for?

I am very much a believer in doing whatever makes you feel your best self. Nobody should judge what that is or how you acquire it. Each of us is on our own life path and can only ever begin to imagine what others may go through or feel. But I quickly learned that although invasive procedures can be truly brilliant and what we can achieve with aesthetic medicine today is fantastic, there is a dark side, too. The short-lived 'happiness' clients experienced on seeing results came at a deep internal cost: an expectation of perfection that doesn't exist, creating, in turn, insecurities that were not there to begin with. Of course, the aesthetic industry is not entirely to blame, as social media and societal pressures all play a part, but for me? I was beginning to see that a more 'natural' approach felt safer, both physically and mentally.

So I went full circle and came back to what I knew and loved: non-invasive and natural treatments to help enhance already beautiful features. And this time it was about focusing fully on the power of hands with something that has been around for centuries – deep-tissue massage for the face and simple facial exercises. Techniques I knew, adored and had been offering for years, only now, more focused and defined. Realising that my true passion was for education within the industry, I continued to empower my clients, as well as other practitioners, reminding them of the beauty of our natural features and sharing the wonder of facial massage with brands across the globe.

My own skin journey

My mother taught me at a young age about holistic therapies and the wonderful benefits they offer. I have fond memories of us learning about alternative medicine together – things like homeopathy and acupuncture, in which I still see great value today.

My mother also taught me how important it is to love and have faith in ourselves and our bodies, and to learn to embrace our uniqueness. She believed we should treat every day as the beautiful gift it is, because tomorrow is never guaranteed – and for that I'm forever grateful.

When it comes to internal health, I suffered with stomach issues, such as sickness, bloating and pain, from a very young age. Neither my parents nor the doctors could find answers, putting it down to me simply being a poorly child. As I got older and began to venture into this industry, I met more and more medical professionals, and started researching the area myself. This included nutritionist visits, food-intolerance tests and experimenting with cutting out certain food groups to try to identify the cause. And I'm still learning; it's always a journey. But it wasn't until my skin became another tell-tale sign that I really committed to keeping up with my gut-health practices. The saying 'you are what you eat' couldn't be more true – whatever is going on internally can – and will – absolutely show up on your skin, the body's largest organ.

Enter perioral dermatitis (PD) – the skin condition some of us have the dubious pleasure of experiencing, with itchy, flaky red bumps around the nose and mouth. Sounds delightful, doesn't it? And those who understand the frustrating nature of this skin condition will know just how confusing it is to treat. Much like other skin conditions – acne, eczema, psoriasis, rosacea, to name a few – PD has a strong link with gut health. The gut is said to be a second brain, and when I first experienced this skin condition, in my mid-20s, I knew there had to be a direct link.

From my work with multiple skincare products and treatments, I was confident that I knew what my skin needed in order to look and feel its best day to day – and that was minimal fuss. I knew my skin had the tendency to be more sensitive, showing up with breakouts from time to time, and that I needed a consistent, simple routine.

Although my PD was mild, it was another reminder of just how incredible the human body is, as mine was clearly giving me a hint about what was happening internally. While I don't necessarily believe in restricting entirely the things we enjoy – life is too short – this was another reminder that perhaps I wasn't paying enough attention to my diet and what my body needed. So I made sure I was following routines that I knew worked for me and my body, such as supplementing with probiotics daily to maintain a healthy gut balance and limiting the amount of yeast in my diet, as that proved to be a huge trigger (of course, everything containing yeast has to be the most delicious!). Although it can be debilitating to suffer from a skin condition that you can't just treat in a matter of days or clear with a new AHA serum, PD ignited a strong interest in, and passion for, finding the root cause for such conditions, rather than treating them with a plaster fix. So I built on my knowledge, spoke to professionals in my field and dug a little deeper. In the beauty industry you are always learning as new technologies and research move on.

I still have occasional flare-ups (around one a year), but these are much more manageable now, although PD is something I will live with for ever. All the practices and advice in this book will help to manage PD, but I have included more tailored advice on pp. 55–57 for this and other conditions.

My community

The best part of developing in any line of work is being able to share the knowledge you acquire with others. For me, recognising how much I can help people daily is extremely rewarding, especially in times of hardship, and if there was one particular time when we all needed support from every which angle, lockdown 2020 was it. This was a time when the beauty industry in particular struggled greatly; a time when creativity was the key to survival for brands; and when pivoting to a focus on digital was very much the answer. Webinars, Instagram lives and Zoom calls were used to build communities all over the world, bringing a sense of peace and a new normality to difficult times. I always think about how much more alone some of us would have felt without social media.

This was also a time when I personally got to share my passion and professional knowledge globally, reaching more people than I ever imagined possible. Unable to visit their regular facialists or local practitioners to help them look and feel their very best, many people turned to the internet to learn how to perform techniques at home themselves. It was incredible to see the engagement of so many, as people from all around the globe came to my sessions to learn natural facial techniques they had previously never heard of but were keen to learn and spread the word about. Many had an awareness of facial massage or exercises, but were unsure how to practise them correctly, and this made me even more eager to spread my expertise. How to define the jawline, enhance the cheeks, lift the brows, open the eyes – you name it, there was a technique to pass on.

With knowledge and positivity being shared, of course the results came pouring in, and so my online community grew. I'll never forget the many messages I would wake up to. It truly gave me drive, motivation and purpose at an otherwise incredibly sad time. One message I'll always remember came from a lovely lady who reached out to tell her story about an illness and medication that caused her face to swell and feel puffy daily. Since practising my techniques at home, her face has returned to its pre-illness state. Her exact words were: 'I can't believe how much they've changed my face, I'm feeling so much better and more confident – I feel like myself again! Thank you so much for putting the sessions on!' It was incredible feedback, and I have saved this and other wonderful messages to remind myself this is why I do what I do, and that this is where my community started.

To this day, the community is growing and growing. That's the wonder of social media and what it should be used for. It's not easy to find like-minded people or make new friends on a daily basis, which is why this platform is so powerful. It's about building new connections and sharing passions with others, wherever you are.

If you want to join the online community, **www.sophieanneperry.com** is where you will find us. And I cannot wait to meet you.

This book

There are so many positive elements to social media, but there will always be negatives, too: heavy screen time being right up there, preventing our brains from fully relaxing and switching off. It's also great at providing a snapshot but doesn't always give people the specifics I like to get across.

So this book is a space in which I can give you a detailed overview of what you should be doing and why.

It is an extension of my community. And it is here to remind you to carve out time in your hectic schedule – time away from screens, time for you to recharge, reflect and unwind.

My values

Now, before we get started, I just want to outline a couple of points that are key to my outlook on beauty.

THE PRIVILEGE OF SKIN AGEING

With the privilege that is ageing, certain natural changes take place within the skin. I'll discuss the biology in more detail in the next chapter, but it's the collagen and elastin fibres in our skin that keep it taut and supple, and with the natural process of ageing, these begin to decline in number, meaning the skin does not appear as plump as it once was (I refuse to use the word 'sag' here, as it just sounds so negative). This can manifest on the face in the form of fine lines and wrinkles from repetitive muscle action, such as forehead lines from frowning or laughter lines around the mouth (or 'memory lines', as I prefer to call them). The skin can also be affected by reduced water content, leading to a drier complexion, or by the muscles in the face becoming weaker and losing their firmness.

These are all natural changes, yet we've been programmed to believe that we need to prevent them in order to continue looking beautiful. But they cannot be prevented indefinitely (nor should they be), and although we can play a part in controlling the rate at which they occur through healthy lifestyle choices and the practices in this book, ageing is a beautiful part of life. And the sooner we get on board with this concept and change the narrative – and by 'we', I mean the industry itself, as well as all of us as individuals – the more beautiful the journey will be in every sense.

BEAUTY FROM WITHIN

'Beauty from within' is a phrase with so many meanings attached to it. Yes, what we eat absolutely has a direct impact on our bodies and can be highlighted through our skin, but let's take a step back. What 'beauty from within' truly means to me is feeling comfortable within yourself and allowing your true self to shine out – something that I believe this industry has somewhat lost sight of.

It can be so easy to fall into the comparison trap of unrealistic expectations of perfection, especially when those expectations are seen through a filter or airbrushed photo on someone's highlight feed on Instagram. We've all been there, scrolling through photos on social media, feeling negative about ourselves based on images of others. But true beauty isn't a look – it's a *feeling*. How we feel about ourselves, and the positive thoughts and words of affirmation we say about ourselves radiate, creating, in turn, a healthy physicality. As my family has always said, 'Your mental state dictates your physical state'.

The ancient techniques in this book act as a form of relaxation and self-care – a way of unwinding, not dissimilar to practices such as yoga or Ayurveda (meaning 'knowledge of life' – a natural system of medicine originating in India), which encourage balance between body, mind and spirit, to bring about a sense of harmony in life.

Facial practices, including the likes of acupressure (where manual pressure is applied to specific 'acupoints'), involve movements to help rebalance energy pathways, as well as deep, rigorous massage to stimulate the muscles and underlying tissues, improving the health and condition of the skin. Combining these techniques and applying them daily to help tackle stress, calm the nervous system and promote a healthy mental state – that, to me, is beauty from within.

So with all that said, and without further ado, let's move on to the knowledge! I hope the next section will empower you with the understanding of how our wonderful bodies function, so you can work with your skin to achieve the results you want. Our skin truly is incredible and the following section explains why it so deserves to be loved and taken care of.

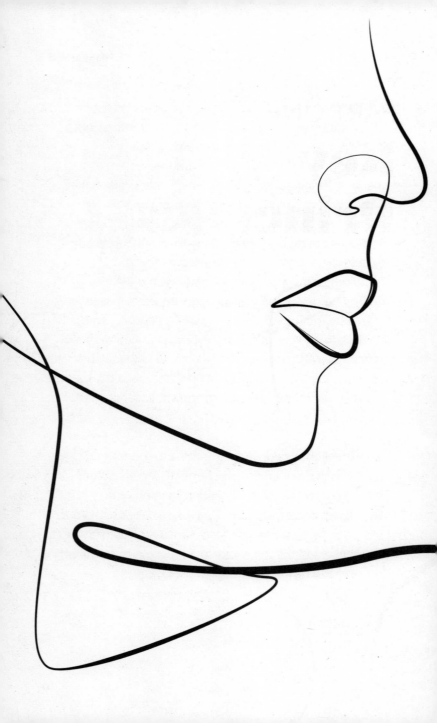

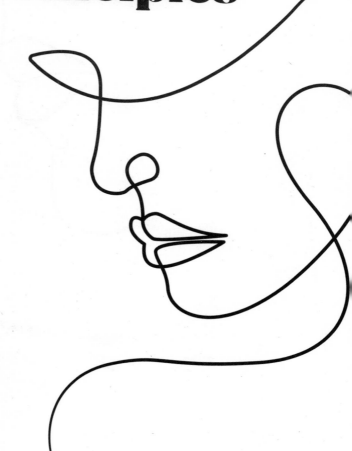

PART ONE

Key Principles

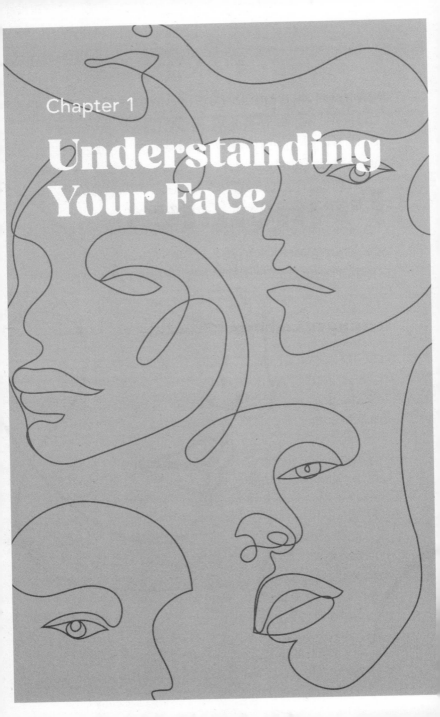

Chapter 1

Understanding Your Face

Before we dive into the practices themselves, I think it's super helpful to understand a bit about the skin and what lies beneath it. You are much more likely to stick with any facial regime if you have this knowledge and are mindful of the structure of your face. That's why this chapter unpacks the science behind what you see when you look in the mirror and how you can harness this for the best possible results.

Getting to know your muscles

First things first – I'd like to explain a little about our muscles, both in terms of the important role they play and what they require for optimal health. Once you know this, it becomes clear why the facial practices in this book are so beneficial.

The muscles in the body are made up of long cords known as muscle fibres that bundle tightly together. These bundles receive signals from the nervous system to contract the fibres, which, in turn, generates motion to produce almost all the movements we make. The facial muscles play a vital role in the way we look, as they provide the face's structure and are closely connected to the skin. When they contract, they pull the face into shape, revealing our expressions to the world, both conscious and unconscious. So when we feel stressed it can very much show.

Facial muscles do not attach directly to bone; they delicately intertwine with each other, like muscular spaghetti. If you're feeling particularly tense in one area, therefore, it's likely to have a direct impact on another. The 'stress triangle' is a great example of this, where tension in the neck can radiate up to the jaw and into the head.

Our muscles need oxygen and energy for optimal health, which is provided through repetitive movement. Sounds simple, right? However, when we're stressed, we tend to tense and tighten certain muscles groups, which then restricts the flow of blood, in turn restricting oxygen and nutrients to the muscles. For example, have you ever felt stressed about a deadline and noticed your shoulders up by your ears? Or your posture as you lean over a computer keyboard? The muscles begin to feel stiff and sore, creating what we know as tension knots in the fibres. The best way to release that tension is through movement, and the facial practices in this book are perfect for giving the muscles what they need.

It's incredibly beneficial to get to know your facial muscles in more detail, understanding which you're contracting day to day – most likely more on one side than the other – and in which you might be feeling tension. Or, indeed, where discomfort may be coming from. With this in mind, a great exercise is to practise finding and isolating each muscle group of the face, and discovering what its action is. Let's give it a try...

Meet your muscles

To help you get to know the muscles better, use the instructions over the page to try flexing each one separately. Being able to isolate an individual muscle is key to making sure they're all getting enough attention.

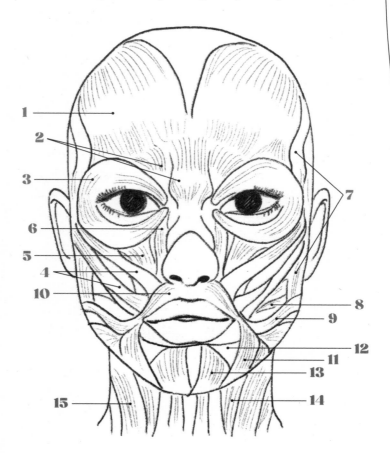

UPPER FACE

1 Frontalis – lift your eyebrows as though in surprise
2 Corrugator supercilii and procerus – draw your eyebrows together in a frown
3 Orbicularis oculi – blink your eyes

MID-FACE

4 Zygomaticus major and minor – create a smile, pulling the mouth upwards and outwards
5 Levator labii superioris – lift each corner of the mouth upwards
6 Levator labii superioris alaeque nasi – lift the upper lip in a snarl
7 Masseter and temporalis – pretend you're chewing a big mouthful of food in an exaggerated manner
8 Buccinator – fill your cheeks with air and purse your lips, like a puffer fish, and blow out slowly
9 Risorius – stretch your lips out horizontally, without lifting the corners upwards
10 Obicularis oris – pout your lips and then relax them, repeatedly
11 Depressor anguli oris – turn the corners of the mouth downwards in an upside-down smile
12 Depressor labii inferioris – stick the lower lip out, like a child about to cry
13 Mentalis – stick the lower lip out even further

LOWER FACE

14 Platysma – pull the corners of your mouth outwards and downwards

15 Sternocleidomastoid – nod your head up and down, then turn your head left and right

Getting familiar with these muscles will make you look at your face in a totally different way – not just the skin you can see, but the many interacting parts. What a marvel it is!

Structure of the skin

As we've seen, the muscles play a key part in what we see in the mirror and, in my opinion, they don't get enough attention. But there are other elements that make up the face, all of which contribute to your health and wellness, as well as your appearance.

Skin is beyond incredible – as mentioned earlier, it is the body's largest organ and one that never ceases to amaze me. Your skin constantly renews itself every 28 days, creating fresh new cells and, in turn, shedding the dead ones. (It's said that humans shed around 600,000 cells per day!) It comprises approximately 16 per cent of your body weight and covers, on average, an area of $2m^2$.

The skin itself has a complex, intricate structure, consisting of three main layers:

THE EPIDERMIS

Your skin's outermost layer – the epidermis – is the thinnest, and is responsible for protecting the body from harm, for new cell development, such as our melanin production (a substance that produces pigmentation in our skin, absorbing harmful UV rays) and keeping the skin hydrated and healthy.

THE DERMIS

The middle layer, or dermis, is the thickest and contains vital structures to support and nourish the skin, such as blood vessels that supply a flow of nutrients and oxygen to the skin, as well as removing waste products. The dermis is home to nerve endings, hair follicles, sweat glands and sensory receptors, just to name a few. It consists mainly of connective-tissue fibres made up of the proteins collagen and elastin. These support the skin's overall form and structure, providing strength and flexibility – something we will look at throughout this book.

THE HYPODERMIS

This is the bottom layer of the skin, connecting the skin to the muscles and bones, insulating the body and storing its energy. The hypodermis is predominately made up of adipose tissue and connective tissue (known as myofascial), providing stability and structure.

Functions of the skin

Our skin is likely to be the first thing people see when they look at us, and we are in the habit of scrutinising our own in the mirror, too. We can spend hours examining pimples, enlarged pores, discolouration or uneven texture, but we forget how many incredible functions the skin has. It's not there just to cover up our insides or make us look good. Let's take a look at some of the other amazing things it does.

PROTECTION AND ABSORPTION

A first line of defence against the environment, the skin cleverly offers its own level of protection from UV light radiating from the sun, with a response system in the form of melanin production. It also creates a physical barrier against any stress, impact, pressure or trauma with flexible collagen fibres, as well as preventing the absorption of harmful substances.

Sebaceous glands located in the dermis produce an oily substance called sebum, which helps keep the skin hydrated and supple, protecting us from moisture loss and dehydration.

The sweat we produce works in unison with the sebum production, forming a protective layer known as our acid mantle, safeguarding us against bacteria overgrowth and fungi and maintaining a heathy skin balance. It's important to understand this, so that we don't overstimulate and compromise our protective barrier with too many resurfacing products or treatments.

As well as protecting, thousands of pores on the surface of the skin can absorb helpful things like vitamins, water and oxygen, needed to provide and maintain a nourished environment. Vitamin D is created by the body on the skin from direct sunlight, aiding the absorption of calcium from the gut, necessary for the health of bones, teeth and nerves. That said, there is a fine line between a healthy amount of direct sunlight being absorbed into the skin and the risks associated with not being adequately protected by an SPF (see p. 41 for more on this).

SENSATION

The skin is home to nerve endings and sensory receptors, detecting stimuli like cold, heat, contact and pain. These nerve endings trigger impulses to the central nervous system, keeping your brain in the loop, so you can respond as necessary to your surroundings – for example, the instinctive response to remove your hand from a hot flame.

Of course, you can also harness the positive sensations that come with gentle touch and massage to relax the nervous system and reduce anxiety or stress – it's all about that mind–body connection.

THERMAL REGULATION AND DETOXIFICATION

Sweat glands and blood vessels aid the skin in regulating the body's temperature. For example, during exercise, the blood vessels dilate to let more blood pass along the skin, allowing heat to be released through the surface. The sweat glands produce perspiration that draws to the surface, then evaporates in an action that cools the body. This is an incredibly sophisticated mechanism our body performs by itself – people usually think of sweat as being gross, but it is actually very useful.

As well as regulating body temperature, sweat glands help to rid us of unwanted toxins, preventing a build-up. I always like to think in terms of 'movement is health, stagnation is disease' – a key topic and one we will come back to shortly.

The lymphatic system

How many times have you woken up from what you thought was a blissful eight-hour sleep (the dream), looked in the mirror and seen a pair of gloriously puffy eyes staring back at you? (Or, indeed, a puffy face in general?) We tend to expect eye circles as a result of a lack of sleep, but not after a good night. But, in fact, during sleep, our bodies switch to relax-and-repair mode, so the rate at which our heart pumps blood through the body slows down. This, in turn, means our lymphatic system naturally slows down, too. So if fluid is being retained and not being flushed out as quickly, it's not surprising that we wake up a little puffy.

The lymphatic system is often referred to as the body's internal irrigation system, removing waste, toxins and excess water – and playing a crucial part in the condition of our skin. It is made up of millions of fine vessels that branch all around the body, carrying a colourless fluid called lymph. Lymph contains white blood cells to help the body fight infection. It also transports waste products and destroyed bacteria back into the bloodstream, ready for removal from the body by the liver and kidneys.

As the lymphatic system doesn't have a pump of its own, it relies on the movement of our muscles in order to flow efficiently. That's why maintaining a healthy lifestyle is so important, as things like poor diet, lack of exercise and even shallow breathing can slow down and restrict the drainage process. If the lymphatic system gets overloaded, you can see the effect in the condition of your skin - with effects including acne, puffy and dull skin or dry patches. Remember: movement is health, stagnation is disease.

Understanding that this particular system doesn't work with a pump to help drain itself means we can begin to see how powerful the art of massage is all over the body, especially the face. The head and neck contain a large proportion of the lymphatic network – more than 300 nodes and channels. Therefore, practising the art of facial massage is key to working with your body's amazing natural systems.

With many of the lymph vessels sitting very close to the skin's surface, minimal pressure or force is required – just consistency and repetition. Lymphatic-massage techniques can be performed across the entire body and, done regularly, your skin will reap the rewards. A healthy, glowing complexion from a healthy, fluid-moving blood flow? Yes please!

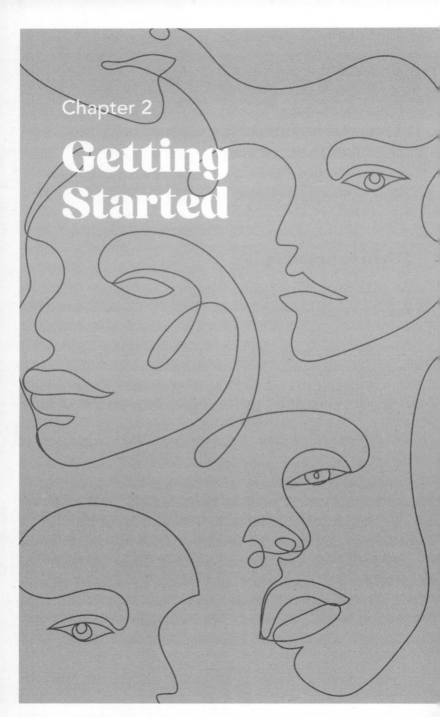

Chapter 2

Getting
Started

Now you know a little bit about the structure of your skin and the support system it sits on, it's time to understand the practicalities of using these techniques. I'll start with a few commonly asked questions.

When to practise

Q. When should I practise my techniques – in the morning or the evening?

A. The short answer here: whenever works best for you. It's always interesting speaking to clients and finding the sweet spot in their routines – whether they like to start their day with a little self-care or whether these facial practices are part of a winding-down process, erasing any negatives from the day and preparing for sleep. Some people prefer to wake up earlier each morning to do the techniques, while others cherish every minute of sleep they can possibly get. Still others prefer not to have a timetable for their facial practices at all, and just fit them in when they can; and while not having a fixed routine can make it harder to remember to do them every day, it certainly doesn't impact their effectiveness.

Forcing yourself to spend ten minutes on your face in the morning when you've got the school run to do or an early start in the office isn't going to provide you with positive benefits, either physically or mentally. It's only going to add more stress to your day and make you resent doing the techniques. So if you know you have more time to dedicate to yourself in the evening, then that's your time. As I said, it's whatever works for you. And the beauty of this is that it gives you more reason to carve out that precious time for you.

For me, it's the morning. I thrive on getting some movement in to start the day, either in the form of a run or a HIIT class, or sometimes with a full-body stretching sequence or 20 minutes of Pilates. Don't get me wrong, it's not always easy (and I don't manage it every morning), but once I've done it, I feel like it's set the tone for the rest of the day. And without fail, my facial techniques follow – a full-body wake up and energise.

Now if you're thinking that all this just sounds like more to add into your already crazy, manic life, I should reassure you that it takes less time than you think. We will talk about the length of time you should spend on your face shortly, but the goal here is consistency – finding your 'when' and creating a ritual you know you'll keep up with. The best advice I can give you is simply to try to do a little every day; you can absolutely see results from just five minutes a day.

What to use

Q. Don't the techniques pull and tug at the skin, causing more facial wrinkles and fine lines?

A. When you're new to this world, it makes perfect sense to ask this question. Depending on the technique, for massage, the rule of thumb is as long as you're using a product on the face that creates slip and glide on the skin, you will be causing zero harm and only doing good, as you're working that little bit deeper, much like a body massage. We are taught to lightly pat our products in, but to improve skin health we need to be working them into the skin.

Some exercise techniques in this book are best done without product, as they're focused on breaking up blockages in the fascia tissue, and it's easier to grip and manipulate these without product. I will highlight which require just clean skin and hands, but the majority of the massage-based practices do require a product of some sort – something that adds a slip and glide to the skin being the goal. As with a body massage again, you need something that allows for a full range of motion without causing too much friction and tug to the skin.

Where a face oil or similar product is required, you will see this icon:

Q. So what's the best product to use?

A. This very much depends on your skin's needs and the time you have to focus on your practice. But I always like to recommend an oil-based product, as this allows time to massage without absorbing into the skin too quickly.

Many of us have a fear of oil-based products, as we've been programmed to believe that oily or combination skin types shouldn't be using them. But oily skin can absolutely benefit from using oils – in fact, products that try to eliminate oil are more likely to overstrip your skin's barrier, leading to more sebum production to compensate, making you even more oily.

It's best to lean towards an oil that acts as an emollient, penetrating deeper into the skin. I've found natural oils, such as pure jojoba, squalene and sea buckthorn oil or products containing these ingredients, to be brilliant, repairing the skin's barrier and keeping it hydrated without sitting on top, creating that oily sheen. For oily skin, a non-comedogenic product (one containing ingredients that will not block your pores), free from artificial colours, preservatives and fragrances is great, as it needs the moisture and nourishment.

You can apply your oil-based product as part of your morning regime, after cleansing and toning, energising the skin before finishing with your moisturiser and SPF. Or it can be great as part of the last step in your night-time routine, either before or after moisturiser (now there's a topic for debate!). A nourishing, nutritious oil to perform your practice at bedtime acts as a real treat for the face before it repairs overnight.

For those who like to follow their routine in the morning but struggle to allow time for it to fully sink into the skin, an option can be to add massage into the cleansing routine (my own solution). You can use your cleanser as a facial massage oil, so perform the massage while cleansing. This is great for those who are still wary and on the hunt for their perfect oil companion, as they prefer the sense of washing off the cleanser and it slowly introduces the ingredients into the routine.

There are also many incredible, lightweight oils on the market with a consistency more like a serum, which is a great option for a morning routine, conferring the benefits of an oil, while sinking into the skin in minutes.

Again, it's a question of finding what works best for you and fits into your routine well. I switch it up from time to time, as skin changes like the seasons, depending on all sorts of life factors. So I might create a window for an evening routine a couple of times a week, which gives me time to extend my practice and enhance the results. I also find it the best way to destress from a difficult day.

Your daily skincare routine

Maintaining a consistent daily skincare routine is important in boosting your skin's health, allowing it to maximise its ability to renew, repair, protect and regenerate. It doesn't need to be complicated – just make sure you're sticking to the core pillars and are staying consistent:

CLEANSE

This is one of the most important steps in any and every skincare routine. Our skin repairs while we sleep, therefore a nightly cleanse to remove the day, and all the dirt and pollution that come with it, is essential for a healthy complexion. There are many cleansers on the market to choose from, so it's important to look for the right one for your skin type. Balms or oil cleansers are my preference; they make it easy to add in facial practices as part of the cleanse and are great for all types of skin.

I'm not one to preach about the need for a full cleanse twice daily, though, as we can absolutely overdo it, compromising the skin's protective barrier. For a morning cleanse, I keep it minimal, unless I'm working out in the morning or have been using an active product during the night that requires a full-face cleanse to remove it. A miscellar water (a cleansing water that's readily available in chemists) is a great option to prep and wake up the face first thing, and many contain ingredients such as salicylic acid, which is great for combination skins.

Something you could consider is an oil cleansing method – I love to recommend this for an oily, acne-prone, perhaps inflamed skin. It means cleansing with a pure oil and then applying again to moisturise, using nothing but this one product (one with natural ingredients, such as sea buckthorn). This acts as a reset for the skin, restoring and rebalancing it to its natural form.

TONE

There are differing views about this step in a regime, but I think it is important for enhancing the cleanse, so if you are prone to more of an oily, congested skin, it's a great addition for removing impurities. More importantly, though, it is also an opportunity to flood the skin with the hydrating ingredients it needs, so dry skin can absolutely benefit from this step.

For my skin (combination), I like to use an essence toner or mist, helping to replenish, balance, hydrate and nourish, prior to applying active serums – rather like a drink for the skin.

SERUM

Serums are such a valuable step in a routine, predominantly applied in the morning due to the ingredients, but you can find many night-time active serums that work really well for an overnight exfoliation. Serums are packed with larger amounts of active ingredients that are easily received by the skin. The lightweight consistency allows them to better penetrate the layers and, given their higher concentration, results can be seen fairly quickly.

I like to describe serums as add-in solutions for any and every situation. For example, if you want to target a specific need, such as hyper-pigmentation or fine lines, a serum with certain active ingredients (such as vitamin C or ceramides) is transformational, while layering or cocktailing a few serums together is beautiful. I'm a serum junkie and will layer at least two of a morning.

Another benefit of serums is that the fast-absorbing delivery system means the face isn't left with a heavy sheen. Applying serums packed full of antioxidants such as vitamin C in the morning is super beneficial in helping to protect the face for the day.

EYE CREAM/SERUM

The skin around the eyes is up to 40 times thinner and more fragile than on the rest of the face – therefore, in my opinion, it's very worthwhile to use a dedicated product to help nourish and soothe this area, as well as protect it. I'm always asked whether it's an essential step in a routine and my answer is no, it's not, and yes, your regular serums will work up to and around this area. However, just as you might target a specific area, such as your abs, when you work out, and that means practising specific movements, the eye area is delicate and benefits from a more targeted product to help tighten, hydrate and treat common skin needs. Face serums can be incredibly active, as I said, so choosing a product tailored specifically for this area is advisable. I also like to do a mini eye massage when applying.

MOISTURISER

This is the step that seals it all in.

Let's start by noting that dry skin lacks oil and dehydrated skin lacks water. Typically, water-based (although some contain oil) moisturisers – as the name suggests – are like a drink for the skin. They help to top up and replenish the skin's water content, but, most importantly, they help it to hold on to it. I like to say that they lock everything in. And as we're applying all these wonderful active ingredients to help our skin flourish, we want to make sure it can keep hold of them.

And what about face oils? Face oils are like a superfood for the skin, and dry skins definitely benefit from this addition. They too work by sealing everything in, ensuring water content isn't lost, but also protecting the skin's barrier by repairing and nourishing it with enriched ingredients. So if your skin is feeling particularly thirsty (dry, tight or dull-looking), a face oil is a great option, either instead of or as well as your moisturiser. I personally opt for applying both of an evening due to the consistency and the fact that it can spend longer on the skin overnight.

SPF – MORNING ONLY

Enter sun protection! As discussed earlier, our skin works with its own clever level of protection, and sunlight can be beneficial to it, as well as boosting general health and wellbeing. However, overexposure is incredibly damaging, and our skin cannot, unfortunately, protect us enough from all the environment has to offer. SPF defends against factors such as UVA and UVB rays, which harm the skin and cause premature skin ageing. While the worry of ageing per se does not concern me, damaging the health of the skin is a different matter.

UVB rays make up a small percentage of solar radiation, are responsible for causing sunburn and are the leading cause of skin cancer. UVA rays make up the rest, and typically penetrate the skin more deeply, playing a greater role in premature skin ageing. This is a problem all year round, which is why you'll hear industry professionals talking about the need to wear sunscreen every single day, not just when the sun is out. Yes, even in winter!

I'm a big fan of mineral sunscreens as they don't use chemicals like oxybenzone and octinoxate, which may be responsible for disrupting hormone levels in the body. There is also an increased chance of skin irritation with chemical sunscreens, which is not ideal for sensitive skin and skin conditions, plus they take up to 20 minutes to start working post-application. Mineral options offer great protection, as they create a physical barrier between you and the sun upon application. A minimum of SPF 30 is the gold standard.

Some cosmetics contain SPF, but not usually enough for adequate protection, so it's best to use a dedicated sunscreen product. Many also sit on the skin beautifully and provide a very welcome glow. Make-up should be applied after you've added your sunscreen.

During the summer months, a mineral SPF spray is a great addition for topping up protection during the day – and don't forget the scalp.

The practices in these pages all slot into the daily routine I've just outlined – once again, it's a question of finding the time that suits you. Is it during a cleanse or product application in the morning? Or in the evening when you have more time for a wind-down routine with your favourite face oil? Either way, this book is here to help you understand just how simple they are to fit into your day. So why not play around with different times and routines, and discover what works best for you and provides the most benefits?

Enhance your routine

I will forever preach – and I have already said – that our hands are our most valuable tools in this line of work. However, there are also what I like to call 'enhancements' that are incredibly worthwhile.

So where should you start with the variety of facial tools on the market? It can seem overwhelming and difficult to understand what's best for which skin need – the *gua sha* stone vs jade roller, EMS vs micro current, blue vs red LED ... And one practitioner may recommend something very different from another.

My advice would be to keep it simple. Our brains and skin react in a similar way here: overcomplicate things and they will get stressed, and then the tool in question will just sit in the bathroom drawer. So focus on the key goal at hand to identify whether the addition of a tool is right for you, and which would be the best one. Here is a little guide to help you.

MANUAL FACIAL TOOLS

As I keep saying, you absolutely do not need to spend lots of money on fancy equipment to see amazing results. I'm just providing a short guide to the most effective tools out there, so that you can explore if you're interested. Many do have noticeable benefits, but they are not essential for boosting the health of your skin.

Gua sha

A great place to start if you're looking to elevate results is with the beautiful traditional Chinese healing practice of *gua sha* (meaning to rub or scrape stagnation or heat trapped in the body).

Flat, smooth-edged stones, usually made from jade or rose quartz, are worked over the skin to relax tissues and promote detoxification. Traditionally, they were used on the body to treat tight muscles and pain by applying pressure with the tool, and often result in redness and bruising as you heal. Facial *gua sha* adopts the same principles but is much less aggressive – you definitely shouldn't experience bruising.

As I said earlier, we need to approach our faces with the same mentality as we do the body, noticing where we are experiencing stress or tightness. *Gua sha* stones provide additional support to hug the muscles, isolate tension and release the surrounding fascia tissue that may be interfering with or blocking the circulatory system. The result is firmer, smoother, more radiant skin, defined contours and less puffiness.

As the practice of *gua sha* has progressed, many have drawn connections between elements in nature and the tool itself, such as the belief that particular precious stones and crystals have the ability to positively charge the body in different ways – healing, protecting and balancing energy. Popular choices include the following:

* **Green jade** Regarded as the ultimate and most valuable gemstone in traditional Chinese medicine, this is believed to carry a healing energy to restore and rebalance, helping with inflammation and redness. This stone is said to support peace, tranquillity and eternal life.
* **Dark green nephrite** One of my favourites, this is believed to help strengthen the nervous system. It is a powerful stone for protection.
* **Rose quartz** This stone is associated with love and compassion, and with comforting healing properties.
* **White jade** A translucent white stone and a symbol of heaven, this is said to bring peace, clarity and harmony and assist with the body's natural healing processes.
* **Stainless steel** Medical-grade stainless-steel *gua shas* are becoming popular with experts, the benefits being that they are highly durable, easy to grip and can be easily sanitised. They are also self-cooling and more eco-friendly.

I personally prefer to use stainless-steel tools for the body and healing stones for my face. I have an array of different *gua sha* stones that I use – I adore them!

Jade rollers

Jade rollers are also a popular choice, and one that clients often use as an introduction to these practices. I find that they can really only target lymphatic drainage and circulation, as well as providing that cooling touch to the face, whereas with *gua sha*, the angle of the stone means it can reach less accessible parts of the face for a deeper, more purposeful release in all senses. But the jade roller is a more approachable method if you're new to the concept.

ELECTRICAL FACIAL TOOLS

Now this is where I geek out x100, trialling new tech! There are many electrical devices on the market, all boasting similar benefits, so it can be a bit overwhelming to try and choose between them. Here are just a few for you to consider:

Micro-current

You've likely heard of this technology, which has been around for a long time, but has now evolved into impressive at-home versions. These tools use an electrical current to stimulate the tissues.

In my experience, micro-current devices are fantastic for more superficial skin stimulation, generating the healthy flow of blood and oxygen that we love, and creating a more radiant, glowing complexion.

EMS

If you're just looking to buy one electrical facial tool and want quick results, I would recommend this technology, as it works a little deeper: EMS (electrical muscle stimulation) does exactly what it says, creating a deep electrical impulse that stimulates contractions in the muscle. Once you feel that deep muscle movement you realise just how strong it is. As I've said, muscles need energy and oxygen to flourish and maintain health, and this tech works each individual muscle that bit harder to improve its tone and form.

Some at-home EMS face tools are tailored to specific areas, so users can spend more time and attention on the parts they want to, while others work across the entire face. And, of course, done consistently, firming the muscles will boost the health and firmness of the skin. This style of technology is perfect for strengthening the structure of the face, providing a healthy base and foundation.

Radio frequency

Another piece of technology I recommend is radio frequency, also a popular treatment in clinics. It is non-invasive and works by boosting the skin's collagen, using heat and a specific frequency to create a collagen cascade within the dermis, stimulating the fibroblast cells for plump, firm-looking skin. It feels like a hot-stone massage for the face, so is also incredibly relaxing. If you want an in-clinic experience, I'd suggest a course of at least six sessions to start with, due to the fact collagen takes time to regenerate. But there are some great at-home devices, too, available at a lower strength, which is great for maintaining results.

The clear difference with this piece of tech is that it focuses specifically on the health of the skin. We know the dermis is where lots of the magic takes place, and this treatment targets exactly that.

LED

One of my all-time favourites, LED stands for light-emitting diode and is a non-invasive treatment that generates various wavelengths of light and energy to be absorbed into the layers of the skin for a wide range of benefits. Interestingly, it is said that NASA originally developed the technology for plant-growth experiments, later realising the effect it had on wound healing and regeneration. It is one of the simplest at-home treatments and, again, a great place to start if you are new to all this.

LED is widely used among skin experts to increase cell turnover, regenerate the skin and soothe a wide range of skin conditions, such as eczema and acne. The two most common frequencies used in the industry are the red and blue wavelengths. Red focuses on the stimulation of collagen to improve the appearance of fine lines, wrinkles and hyper-pigmentation. Blue is used for its anti-bacterial benefits, killing acne-causing bacteria and reducing the amount of oil that the glands produce within the skin.

There are many at-home versions to choose from, and I always recommend the option of the two frequencies. A flexible mask that provides full coverage of the face and neck is best (there are even options for the body, too). But you should note that the results with LED are not as fast as with the other devices listed here, and patience and consistency are required. You should allow 30 minutes a few times a week to lie still with the mask on. I usually pop on a podcast and detach from the world during treatment.

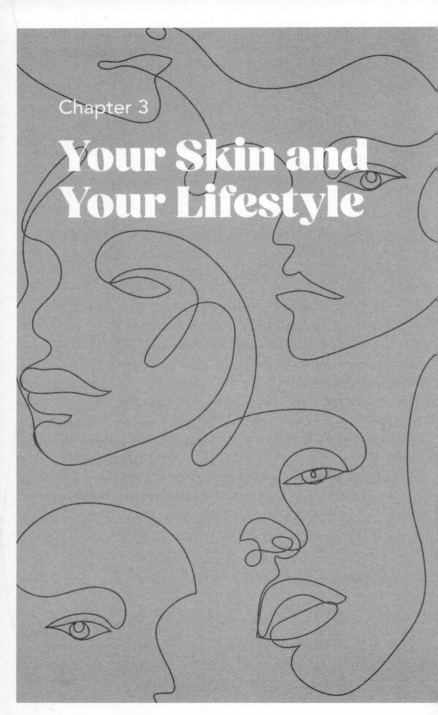

Chapter 3

Your Skin and Your Lifestyle

Facial practices are only one part of maintaining healthy skin. It's vital that you also look at how your lifestyle can impact your skin and what you could incorporate to support everything else you're doing. This chapter will look at some of the key pillars of a healthy lifestyle, as well as what you can do if you have an underlying skin condition.

Diet

Aim for a balanced diet, rich in fruits, vegetables, whole grains (such as oats and quinoa) and lean proteins (skinless chicken, fish, eggs, tofu or tempeh), to provide essential nutrients for healthy skin. For myself, I always prefer plant-based options.

A diet high in processed foods, sugars and unhealthy fats may contribute to skin issues, but they are not always easy to cut out entirely – finding the balance that works for you is key.

Juices are a wonderful way to up your intake of vegetables. I opt for a green juice in the morning, with the addition of celery, that being a favourite for skin health. When I drink this consistently, I notice huge benefits.

Supplements

While a good diet is the best way to get the antioxidants and minerals you need, supplements can help to make sure you're covering all bases. There are some on the market that specifically target healthy skin and hair, but the key things to look out for are vitamins C, D and B7, as well as selenium and omega-3 fatty acids. Collagen supplements have also gained popularity as they can help to improve skin elasticity when used consistently. Looping back to the gut-health factor here, I highly recommend pre- and probiotics to help maintain a heathy gut-flora balance. You can find many options in liquid and capsule form. Always check with a health professional when choosing supplements in case they interfere with other conditions and/or medications.

Hydration

Proper hydration is crucial for maintaining skin health. In addition to applying hydrating products topically, drinking an adequate amount of water (2–3 litres daily) helps to keep the skin fully hydrated, boosting the lymphatic system and flushing out toxins.

Alcohol and caffeine should only be drunk in moderation, as they can dehydrate the skin.

Sleep

This one is tricky, as most of us cannot control the amount of sleep we get, and often, the more we think about it, the more difficult it is to nail down. But bad sleep can really impact the skin. We repair while we sleep, and our skin needs that rest and repair to function optimally.

If you're struggling with sleep, it's worthwhile looking into ways of building healthy routines – such as implementing facial practices as part of your evening wind down. I've found many natural supplements can work wonders here (magnesium has helped me), as well as breathing techniques and meditative sounds (see Resources, p. 150).

I would also like to take this opportunity to recommend that you invest in a silk pillowcase – these are amazing at reducing skin creases and wrinkles, and are also known to help with skin conditions, as they create less friction on your delicate skin and stop it drying out.

Stress

This is another one I don't like to dwell on too much, as no one actively chooses to be stressed. But if you're having issues with your skin, it could be a sign that your cortisol (stress hormone) levels are too high. Finding effective stress-management techniques can be beneficial, including – you guessed it – the practices in this book. Some of the most common feedback I get from clients who apply these techniques daily is about feeling more at ease, centred and less stressed.

Sun exposure

Excessive sun exposure can really damage the skin. As discussed earlier (see p. 41), daily SPF is your best weapon against harmful rays and I've mentioned my personal favourites. Sunglasses when it's bright are also useful for preventing squinting, which can deepen lines around the eyes. If you're in a hot climate and outside during the day, a top-up SPF mist is a must.

Smoking

Most of us know that smoking accelerates ageing and impairs blood circulation, so if you're looking for a reason to quit, perhaps this could be the one. I hope it is!

Exercise

Regular exercise improves blood circulation, which helps to beautifully nourish the skin. It also helps to manage stress levels by releasing endorphins, promoting a healthy, glowing complexion. Any movement at all can benefit the skin, so just find what you like doing – and do it.

Personal habits

I've noticed increasingly that people touch their faces frequently and scrutinise them in the mirror, picking at them physically (popping blackheads, for example) when they feel anxious. If this is you, try to find alternative methods for managing anxiety – perhaps with positive words of affirmation, rather than highlighting flaws. (I also recommend pimple patches to prevent the urge to pick spots.) Other bad habits include not removing make-up before bed and using harsh, quick-fix skincare products that can negatively impact your skin, stripping it of its goodness.

A word on lifestyle and skin conditions

If you suffer from an active skin condition, like high-grade acne, eczema, psoriasis or rosacea, following the advice I've given regarding nutrition and skincare is going to be helpful to you. But here are some additional thoughts that may help during an active flare-up or breakout – or to help prevent them.

NUTRITION

I'm a qualified aesthetician with many different courses under my belt, but I am not a nutritionist and would highly recommend that you find one to help with your specific issues.

I personally try to stick to an anti-inflammatory lifestyle as much as I can – that means vegetables, whole grains, omega-3 fatty acids (found in fish, nuts and seeds, for example) and healthy fats and proteins, while limiting processed foods and sticking to plant-based options.

The candida diet is also super helpful, cutting out sugars, gluten and certain types of dairy, while focusing on including healthy proteins, non-starchy vegetables and high-quality oils (good fats). This particular method aims to restore a healthy balance of yeast and bacteria inside your body – like a reset for your gut microbiome (the community of microbes in your gut). There are lots of books out there to help, if this is something you want to try; it's not the easiest diet when you're new to it, but my skin was showing signs of yeast overgrowth (itchiness and red bumps), and it definitely helped from the outset. If I experience a flare-up (because once you've had one, it can come back, depending on your general health), I lean back into more of a reset and candida cleanse. Day to day, I stick to this lifestyle as much as possible, as I feel best when I do: think more energy and mental clarity. But as I said earlier, I don't deprive myself of the things I enjoy when I'm craving them. It's all about balance, right?

TOPICALLY

I've found gentle cleansing products with hydrating ingredients such as aloe, ceramides and hyaluronic acid are wonderful, as hydration is always key. But there are also plenty of ingredients in skincare products (such as cleansers, shampoos, deodorants and even make-up) that can be quite toxic to the skin. As a general rule, it's best to avoid anything containing sulphates, parabens, phthalates and heavy fragrance and very active ingredients like resurfacing acids. These things are more likely to be about enhancing your experience with the product or increasing its shelf life than improving the health of the skin.

Serums and moisturisers containing niacinamide and polyglutamic acid to feed and nourish are the best products to turn to, as they do not disturb the skin's balance and protective functions. My top tip here? For a particularly bad flare, I have found Sudocrem to be a lifesaver ... the tub of dreams. The zinc ingredient works wonders for calming.

Sadly, during a flare-up, adding make-up into the mix can really aggravate a skin condition – again, due to questionable ingredients. At these times, I keep it minimal, with a tinted BB cream and SPF, paying attention to the ingredients, avoiding those listed above.

Dealing with any active skin condition takes an incredible toll on your mental wellbeing. You can feel embarrassed to leave the house at times, thinking your face is a focal point for others – and that stress cycle keeps the condition thriving. It can be very debilitating and lonely but knowing that many people experience these cycles can help, as does hearing tips of what helps others along the way – perhaps through social media or condition-specific forums online.

There may absolutely be times when you feel you need to lean towards a quick-fix option, such as topical steroids (these are on prescription in the UK). I would view these with caution, however, as I have found symptoms can come back with a vengeance post-steroid use. So when I experience my PD flare-ups (which are thankfully now mild and more manageable), I lean into strengthening my practices in ways that I know work for me and looking within for the root cause, as outlined above. And my skin has never been happier for it.

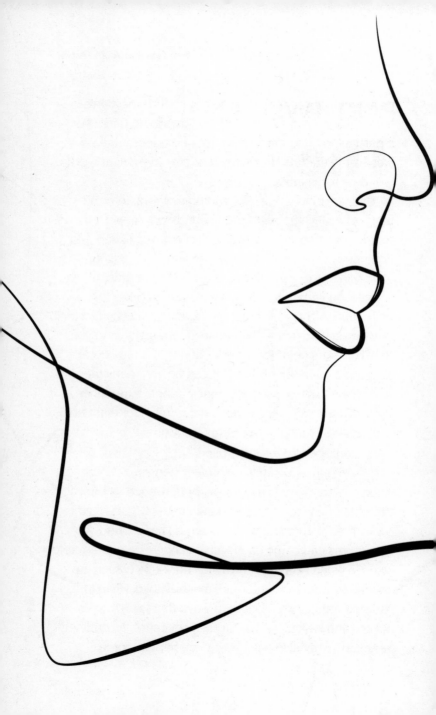

PART TWO

The Practices

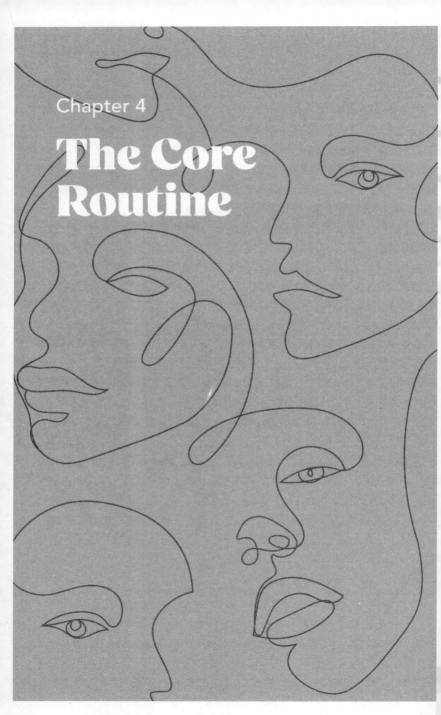

Chapter 4

The Core
Routine

Later on in this part of the book, you'll find that I've isolated specific areas of the face, so that when you feel you'd like to elevate or tweak your daily practice, or personalise it, by focusing more on enhancing the eye area, say, you'll have the relevant techniques to apply.

But it all starts with a core routine: the basis and foundation of your practice – the practice you carve out time in your daily routine to perform. It should be one that simply becomes part of your wellness regime, a daily habit you wouldn't think of skipping. Because the results speak for themselves.

I've designed the following five-minute core routine with simplicity and ease in mind. It is all you need to start achieving the fantastic results detailed in this book, as long as you are consistent and aim to do it every day.

The first time you work through this protocol it may take a little longer, but when you begin to feel confident with the techniques and the sequence, it will become second nature and will not take longer than five minutes.

Once you feel comfortable with your core routine, you may find yourself wanting to add in new techniques to extend your practice. This is where you can start customising, working on different areas of the face and really reaping all the potential benefits. But don't forget, you can still work magic in five minutes if that's all you have!

Before you begin

* Create a self-care space that you feel happy to be in.
* Be sure your hands are clean.
* Select an oil-based product (see pp. 35–37) when prompted. This will enable your fingers to glide over your skin; firm pressure and speed aren't always the answer.
* Check in with yourself and remember that this is your time to relax and be comfortable.
* Take some time for breathwork before you begin if you're feeling particularly stressed – even a few repetitions of breathing in through the nose, holding for four seconds, then breathing out through the mouth will help you to reset and focus. (See Resources, p. 150 for more information.)
* Don't rush – work with intention and stay focused and mindful. You should be able to have fun with it – this is your personal practice, so enjoy it!
* Track your progress: it's not all about the visible benefits, but if you take a clear photo in the same pose (ideally with the same lighting) once a month, this will help to remind you of how far you've come.

Prep

Before beginning any type of exercise regime, preparation is key. This is all about warming up the area, getting the blood and lymph moving, as well as stretching the muscles.

Be sure to watch your breath throughout, focusing on deep inhalations and exhalations; if you catch yourself holding your breath, pause and release. This is important because the lymph works with the breath.

1 **Shoulder rotations** To loosen up the shoulders, sit up straight and slowly roll them in a full circular motion, forwards 5 times and backwards 5 times, opening up the chest and correcting your posture.

2 **Head rotations** Slowly rotate your head round in circular motions, without straining. Repeat 3 times, then repeat another 3 times in the opposite direction.

3 **Neck stretches (side)** Keep your shoulders dropped and posture upright, almost as if there is a piece of string through your head, keeping you upright. Looking forwards, tilt your head slowly to the right, keeping the opposite shoulder down and leaning into the stretch. To intensify, place your right hand lightly on your head behind the ear, allowing the weight of your arm to deepen the stretch, rather than forcing it. Remember to keep the opposite shoulder down and work with the breath. Hold for up to 5 seconds and repeat 5 times before switching sides.

Top tip
With the side-neck stretches, you'll likely feel more tension in one side than the other (perhaps the side you hold a bag on or the side you sleep on); whichever side it is, spend a little more time on that one.

4 **Neck stretch (front)** With your posture upright again, tilt your head back so you're looking up. Place your hands lightly on the chest and feel the stretch at the front of the neck.

Lymphatic focus

Now we're going to activate the key lymph nodes in the face and neck. Remember, the system doesn't have its own pump, so specific movements to wake up different areas are hugely beneficial.

No product is needed here, as this technique utilises light pumping motions across the lymph nodes. And because the lymphatic system can lie close to the skin's surface, this technique isn't all about pressure.

Spend at least 5 seconds on each of the following, remembering to breathe slowly and mindfully.

1 Place your hands under your armpits, fingers pointing forwards and elbows out to the sides. Lightly press the heels of your hands into your armpits and roll the pressure through to your fingers in a wave-like motion. Then swap so that each hand is under the opposite armpit, thumbs out in an L-shape. Repeat this motion.

2 Returning your hands to the starting position, move them inwards, so your fingers are almost touching. Repeat the rolling motion from the step above.

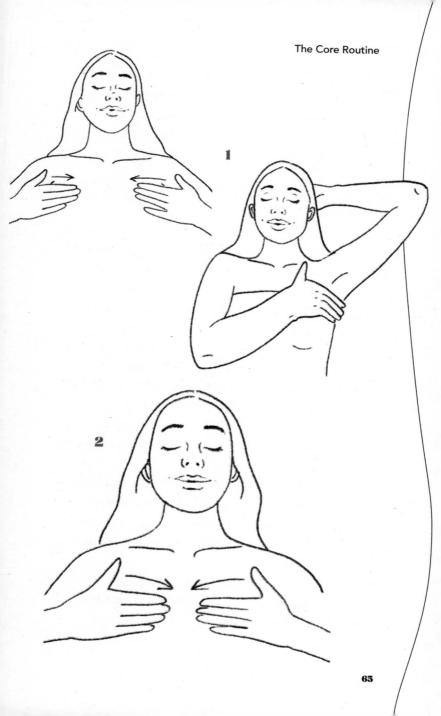

1

2

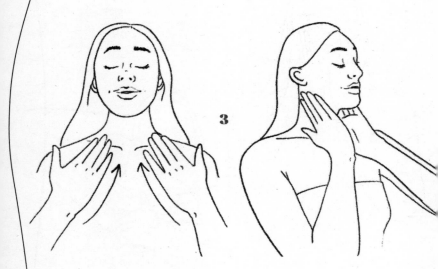

3 Place your hands over your collarbone and repeat the rolling motion from the previous step, then do the same on the sides of the neck.

4 Place your hands on both sides of the face and use the same pumping action from the heel of your hand to your fingertips.

5 I call this move the 'ear Vs'. Paying attention to the groups of lymph nodes around the ear, create a V between your index and other fingers and hook around the ear. Lightly pump in circular motions, encouraging movement through the area.

6 Pump lightly underneath the jawline to the submandibular and submental nodes and back to the ear in a V motion.

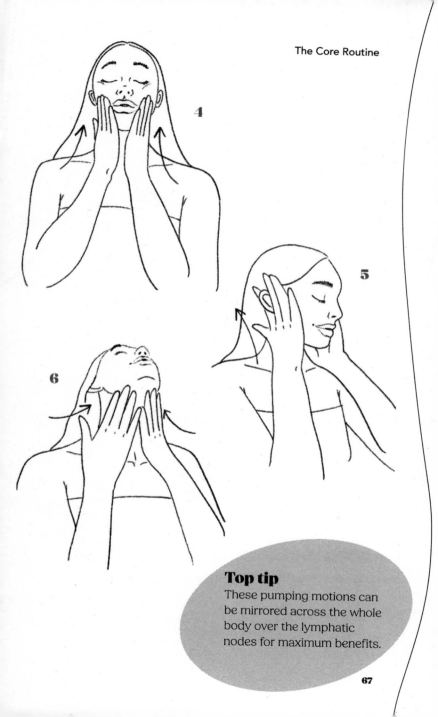

Top tip
These pumping motions can be mirrored across the whole body over the lymphatic nodes for maximum benefits.

STIMULATE

Next up is a focus on bringing warmth through to the tissues, as everything becomes more supple when warm.

Face squats

. . . .

1 Create an O with your mouth, your lips covering your teeth.
2 Place the palms of your hands on your forehead with light pressure only, little fingers covering the eyebrow.
3 Keeping your mouth in the O position, smile and lift the cheeks, holding for 3 seconds; you should feel the cheek area activate. Do 10 contractions, holding each for 3 seconds.
4 Repeat for 3 sets, with only a short gap between each.

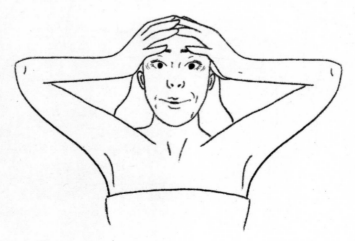

Neck sweeps

1 Apply a reasonable amount of product to the face and neck – start small and add more if needed (it will depend on the type of product you are using, whether it's an oil or a balm).
2 With light pressure, massage in circles on opposite sides of the neck. Repeat 3 times on each side.
3 Create a V shape with your thumbs and fingers, place your hands on opposite sides of the neck at the base of the skull and move your hands down your neck to the collarbone. Repeat 3 times.
4 Place your hands at the back of the neck, so your fingers are touching and slide the hands forwards to flush everything towards the collarbone. Repeat 3 times.

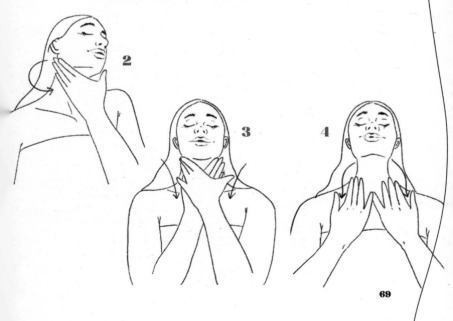

Drainage sweeps

• •

1 Using your full hand and fingers and working on both sides of the face at the same time, use a light pressure to sweep from the centre of the face out towards the lymph nodes at the ear, and down the sides of the neck to the collarbone. Repeat 3 times.

2 Repeat the same motion from the centre of the forehead and down towards the ear, one hand after the other 3 times.

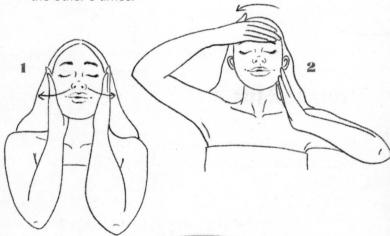

Top tip

If you are pushed for time, make sure the neck gets your full attention. Think of the lymphatic system as a traffic jam – if the neck is blocked, the fluid in the face can't move freely and flourish, so you should work on movement through the neck first.

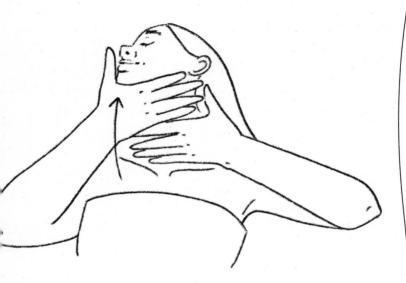

Hug and lift

I like to think of this move as hugging the neck and sweeping upwards, encouraging a lift and stretch to the muscle.

1 With alternate hands use the full palm to mould into the neck and sweep upwards to the jaw with light pressure.
2 Follow with the other hand, as if in one continual motion, working across the full neck, back and forth at least 3 times.

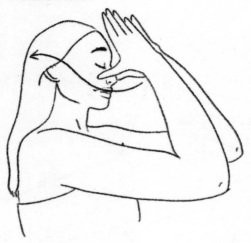

Cheek hug and drain

● ●

1 Put your hands into the prayer position with your thumbs at the corners of your nose and your fingers resting on your forehead.

2 Glide your thumbs, using a medium pressure, contouring under your cheekbones along towards your ears.

3 Finish each movement by sweeping your fingers down the neck from your ears to the collarbone, draining fluid with light pressure.

4 Repeat at least 3 times.

Top tip

When targeting the lymphatic system with a drain, even following a deeper move such as this, always drain with light pressure as a rule.

Upper-face lift

1 Using the middle and ring fingers, begin in the gap between your eyebrows.
2 Press and slide through and above the eyebrows with medium pressure, creating a lift.
3 Lighten off the pressure, moving around and underneath the eyes in a circular motion, reapplying pressure once hitting the eyebrows again.
4 Repeat this move at least 3 times, finishing with a light drain down the face to the collarbone.

Top tip

Under the eye is delicate, so be sure not to apply very deep pressure here. This move can be repeated as many times as needed, especially in the morning, as the area can be prone to poor circulation and puffiness due to the delicate, thin tissue.

ENERGISE

Your face will now be feeling lovely and warm; you may even notice a bright, radiant glow, which is exactly the goal.

The techniques in the Energise section are all about increasing energy production, stimulating circulation and hugely boosting the detoxification process. They are my personal favourites and I always make time for them, no matter what.

Full-face vibrations

1 Separate and open all four fingers on both hands, like a fan.
2 Starting with one cheek at a time, with medium pressure, begin to lift the tissue in a wave-like motion, one hand after the other, creating a ripple effect and wave of vibration across the face.
3 After a few seconds, pick up the pace to really boost circulation, working gradually across the cheek in a back-and-forth motion for at least 30 seconds.
4 Repeat on the other side.

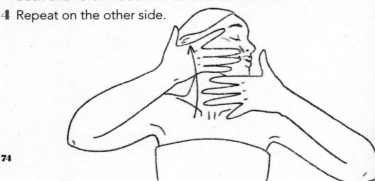

DRAIN

When we stimulate blood and oxygen through the tissues, we also flush through toxins, so it's key to assist in draining these away when we finish our practice. Perform the following final drain techniques at the very end of your core routine.

Final drainage sweeps

1 Using the full hands and flats of the fingers, sweep with light pressure from the centre of the face out towards the lymph nodes at the ears, and down the neck to the collarbone.

2 Work across the forehead, the cheeks and down the neck.

3 Repeat at least 3 times.

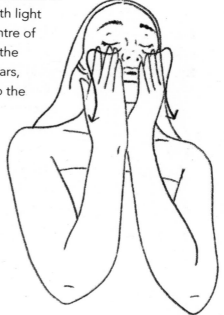

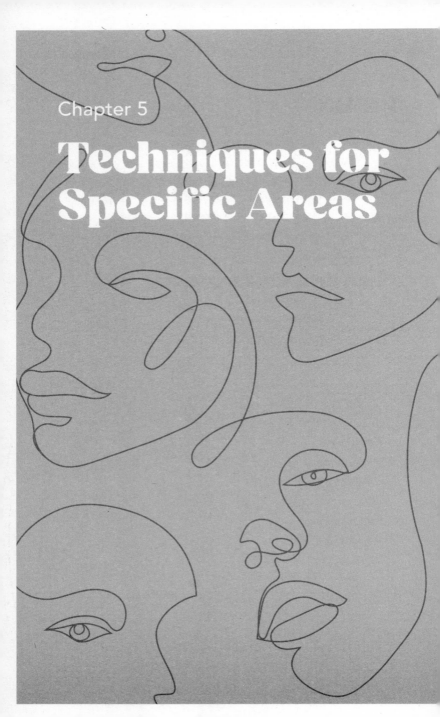

Chapter 5

Techniques for Specific Areas

This chapter is a curation of my best-loved techniques for elevating and enhancing specific areas of the face. Depending on the area you'd like to focus on, just add the relevant techniques to your core routine and create your own bespoke practice, always ending with the lymphatic drainage sweeps (see p. 75).

If you want to elevate your full-face routine, simply add in techniques across all the areas. There are a few options per area for you to choose from. You'll soon find your favourites.

Remember, for exercises that need a face oil or similar product (see pp. 35–37), you will see this icon: 🫙

SHOULDERS AND NECK

Neck strengthening

1 Gently tilt your head back and look at the sky. Now pout your lips sticking your lower jaw out as much as possible (you will feel the platysma muscle working).
2 Hold for up to 5 seconds and repeat up to 5 times.

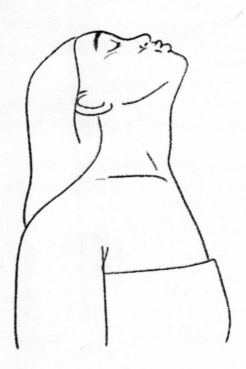

Isolated neck stretches

Correcting your posture throughout the day is important, especially if you work at a screen or use your phone a lot. The platysma is a broad sheet of muscle, responsible for drawing the corners of the mouth down and out, as well as assisting in lifting the head up and down. The skin across the entire neck is also thinner and can benefit from the extra love.

Before moving on to specific techniques for the area I always recommend isolated stretches, extending the prep section. The front of the neck is often forgotten when we think of stretching, and given there are large muscles in the neck, stretching them is super beneficial. This type of isolated stretching also allows you to take note of any areas you feel particularly tense in, spending more time and attention where most needed.

1 Begin by placing one hand underneath the chin and the opposite resting on the collarbone very lightly (this hand helps with resistance).

Top tip
Be mindful of pressure on the collarbone – you want just a light presence here to allow for some resistance to the muscle. Never press firmly on bone.

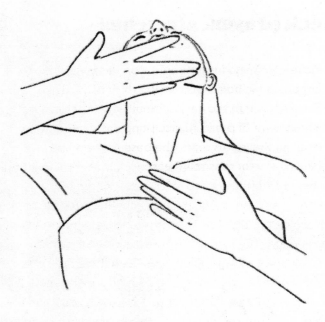

2 Apply pressure with the hand underneath the chin, gradually lifting the head up and back, stretching the front of the muscle. Hold for up to 5 seconds and repeat up to 8 times.

3 Now repeat the same technique, but lean your head to the right rather than backwards. You may need to swap hands, with one underneath the jawbone and the opposite resting gently on the collarbone.

4 Hold for up to 5 seconds and repeat up to 8 times.

5 Lastly, repeat on the left side.

Neck prayer

1 Place your hands together in a prayer position, fingertips facing inwards to the throat.
2 Slowly open up the hands, moulding into the throat with a wave of pressure, sculpting upwards, until the heels of the palms reach the base of the skull.
3 Pause here for tension release.

Top tip

It's important to begin this move with light pressure on the throat, sweeping upwards. Once on the sides of the neck, light to medium pressure can be applied.

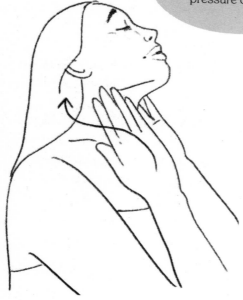

Neck rolling

An intricate technique that appears in some of the other exercises too, this takes a little practice, but provides incredible results. It is a form of myofascial release, working on clearing and releasing obstructions within the soft tissues and improving lymphatic and blood flow, which, in turn, improves the appearance of fine lines.

Make sure there isn't too much product on the face; you'll need hardly any, otherwise you won't be able to grip the tissue. The technique will bring up blood flow and potentially some redness in the skin, which is normal, but never press so firmly that you cause discomfort; the skin here is thin and fragile, so be mindful. Focus on lines you want to improve with this technique – that's what it's great for.

1 With one hand work on the opposite side of the face, starting at the base of the neck in the centre and working your way up.
2 Pinch a small amount of skin between your thumb and your index and middle fingers.
3 Push your thumb towards the back of your neck, allowing your fingers to walk ahead and gather new skin as the thumb glides forwards.
4 Perform up to 8 times per area, if needed, before switching to the opposite side.

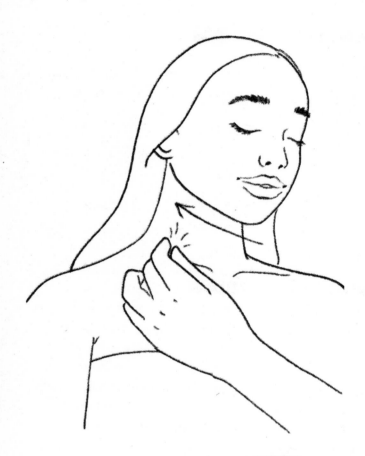

Top tip
Don't rush; this is an intricate technique that requires focus for good results.

MOUTH AND JAW

Clients often ask about these areas. Due to the nature of ageing and gravity, they're parts of the face that many people feel very self-conscious about. The lymphatic channel also runs along and underneath the jawline, so this area can be prone to puffiness (hence the term 'double chin'), in many cases due to fluid retention.

These practices will help to firm and shape the jaw and improve the appearance of laughter lines around the mouth.

Jawline resistance

This move will begin to strengthen the muscles under the jawline, helping to contour the lower face.

1 Make a fist with your dominant hand and rest it underneath your chin. Make sure you're comfortable and your posture is straight with shoulders back and down.
2 Slowly try to open your mouth, lowering your jaw, using your fist while doing so to resist the movement, preventing you from fully opening your mouth.
3 Hold the resistance move for up to 5 seconds, and repeat 5 times.

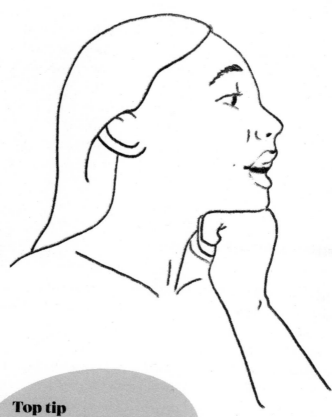

Top tip
Be sure you're not pressing too firmly against your jaw here; you only need light to medium resistance, and shouldn't feel any discomfort.

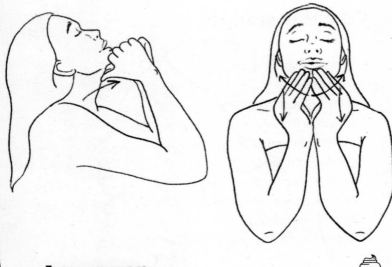

Jaw sweep

This massage technique targets both underneath the jawline and above. It's great for draining excess fluid and defining the area.

1 Place all four fingers of both hands above the chin, with the thumbs sitting underneath.
2 With light to medium pressure, slide along the jawline towards to the ears; we're working along the lymphatic channel here, so I always like to finish each sweep with a drain down the sides of the neck to the terminus. Remember: light pressure for a drain focus.

If this is an area you'd like to enhance, I recommend repeating at least 8 times.

Circular sculpts

1 Working with the same hand and side of your face (i.e. right hand on the right side), use the opposite hand for light support on the chin.

2 Massage in circular motions along the jaw, starting at the chin and ending at your ear, focusing the pressure on the lift upwards, not pulling down. Use medium pressure here with your finger pads. As you're releasing tension above the jawline, the thumb follows lightly underneath it.

3 Repeat up to 8 times before switching sides.

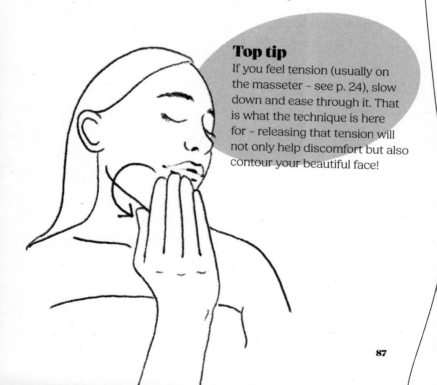

Top tip

If you feel tension (usually on the masseter – see p. 24), slow down and ease through it. That is what the technique is here for – releasing that tension will not only help discomfort but also contour your beautiful face!

Prayer lift and glide

1 Place both hands together in a prayer-like position at the centre of the chin.
2 Slide into the jawline, opening up the hands, moulding them up and along the jawline.
3 Finish a little higher, by the tops of the ears, sculpting, to lift the tissues upwards.

Top tip
Lean into the movement – as the hands open along the face, bow the head down into the move, creating deeper pressure.

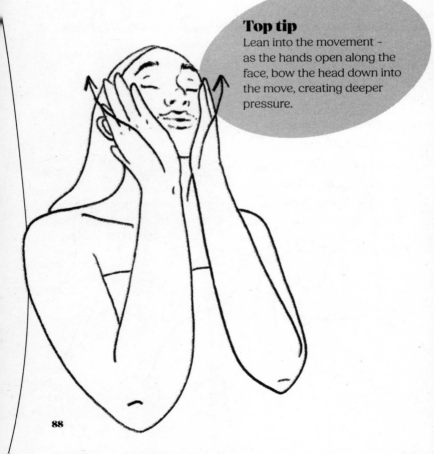

MARIONETTE FOLDS

These are the expression lines that run down vertically from the corners of the mouth. The following techniques help to strengthen the muscles in the lower face and lift the corners of the mouth, drawing the smile upwards.

Lower-face lift

1 Begin by placing your finger pads on your masseter muscle (see p. 24).
2 Lightly lift the skin, pulling towards the ears, keeping it taut.
3 Now blow air out of your mouth 10 times, as if you're blowing out a candle, making an O with your mouth each time.
4 Repeat 20 times.

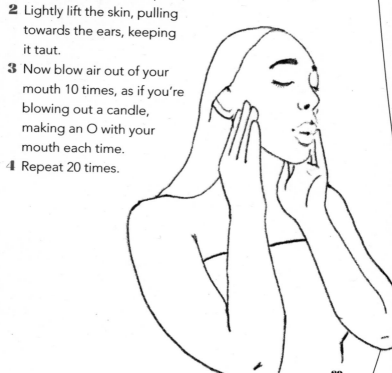

Mini Cs

1 Put your hands in a prayer-like position, palms together.
2 Place both thumbs just slightly underneath your jawline, with your fingertips resting between your eyebrows.
3 Applying medium pressure with the pads of your thumbs, slide them underneath the chin, up towards your marionette folds, naturally transferring the pressure onto the insides of your thumbs as you slide up to the corners of the mouth. At this point, you're lifting the muscle and surrounding tissues up, creating volume almost underneath your cheekbones.
4 Pause for a second and repeat, up to 8 times.

Top tip
Use the full length of your thumbs as much as possible, as this covers the full area, creating more of a lift. Keep the movement slow, feeling for any tension.

Top tip
This move works at lifting up the cheeks, as well as the marionette folds – a technique that can be tailored to many areas of the face.

Repetitive lifts

1 Working on one side at a time, using all four finger pads, lift with medium pressure from the jawline up to the corners of the mouth with one hand.

2 Immediately follow with the other hand. (The goal is to keep the tissues lifted throughout, as one hand follows the other.)

3 Repeat up to 8 times before switching to the opposite side of the face.

LIPS

I am often asked, 'Can you plump the lips with these facial methods?' And the answer is yes, you can, but of course, consistency is needed for good results.

Lip crunches

1 Begin by covering your teeth with your lips (don't force it – just let the lips lightly cover the teeth).
2 Now form what I call a half-smile, drawing your mouth outwards in one long line – you should feel the muscles around the mouth working when holding this position. Your lips may open slightly, which is fine as long as your lips are still covering your teeth.
3 Hold for 2 seconds and relax for 2 seconds. Repeat 20 times.

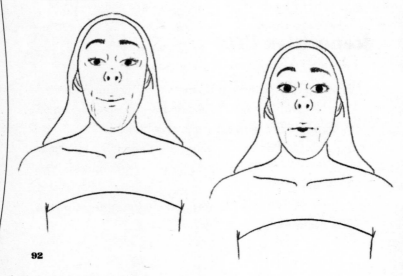

Knead and slide

This technique is all about boosting circulation to the area. If you slip off the muscle continuously, you're using too much product. You need just enough to slide along but not so much that you are unable to grip and hold.

1 Squeeze your lips between your thumbs and middle fingers, by placing your thumbs below your lips and the middle fingers above (you may resemble a duck!). Don't be afraid to really grab on, as this will ensure you're holding the muscle and not just the skin.

2 Squeezing each thumb and finger pair alternately, knead along the lips to one side of the mouth and then back to the other.

3 When you reach the corner of the mouth, you will feel what's called the modiolus (a small ball made up of fibromuscular tissue, where several facial muscles converge). Make sure you are lifting here, not pulling the muscles downwards.

4 Repeat this move back and forth, up to 8 times.

BUCCAL MASSAGE

Enter buccal massage – one of my all-time favourites. 'Buccal' is a term that relates to the cheek and mouth, and buccal massage is an elevated technique that has become widely popular in the industry, and rightly so!

Performed intra-orally, using either a thumb or finger slightly inside the mouth to create a magnet-like effect on the tissues internally and externally, practitioners have been using this technique for many years to help treat conditions such as bruxism (teeth grinding), TMD (temporomandibular disorder, affecting the movement of the jaw), migraines and even Bell's palsy (involving facial muscle weakness or paralysis). I myself suffer with TMD and I know this works wonders.

As discussed earlier, releasing tension in the chewing muscles creates instant contour and definition in the face, and this technique can elevate the results hugely. It can be performed in clinic by a practitioner but can also be done at home and is a valuable addition to your practice.

Below are a few of my favourite buccal massage exercises to try at home. They can be slotted into your practice post-core routine, as buccal massage is a sculpting technique, so it's important to have warmed the fascia, tissues and muscles externally first to make it both comfortable and effective.

I strongly recommend using gloves for this technique, for hygiene purposes; plus, our gums are very delicate, and we don't want to cause any accidental trauma (a scratch with a nail, for example). Nitrile gloves are a good choice, due to the thin material acting like a second skin.

I like to add in some buccal massage to my practice at least once a week – or more, if I'm feeling exceptionally tense.

Buccal massage – some dos and don'ts

* Wear gloves for hygiene and also to protect the sensitive gums.
* When working around shallow areas, such as around the mouth, be sure not to push your thumb too far in the mouth into the gum. Just rest it lightly at the point where you feel resistance.
* This technique is much better with shorter nails.
* Be mindful of the teeth – refrain from resting your thumb on them.
* Apply a lip balm prior to performing the practice to help condition and protect the lips.
* Be sure not to stretch the lips outwards too much, pulling them; once the thumb is inserted, close the mouth.
* Work slowly and feel for tension!

Buccal set-up

1 Add product to your cheeks. Put your gloves on clean hands and ensure your facial tissues are prepped and warm (from your core routine).

2 Begin by working on one side: open your mouth and insert your thumb in the opposite cheek, along the lower gum line, in front of the teeth.

3 Once the length of your thumb is along the gum line, simply close your mouth.

4 Imagine the thumb that's now inside your mouth is glued to one of the fingers on the outside at all points, like a magnet (this is what creates the pressure on the tissues).

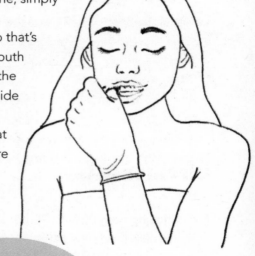

Top tip

The pressure here isn't too firm; light to medium is all that's needed, as it's delicate tissue. And remember, you're only working inside the gum area here; the teeth are always closed for this technique.

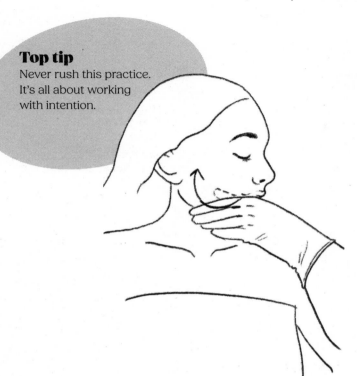

Top tip
Never rush this practice.
It's all about working
with intention.

Circular lifts

1 Continuing from the set-up position, keeping the
   thumb fully inside the mouth, rotate it upwards from the
   marionette folds, in a C-like motion, covering the full
   area, finishing up by the nasolabial folds (the creases
   that extend between the sides of your nose and the
   corners of your mouth). You should complete a full
   circuit of the mid-face, while the flats of all four fingers
   follow externally, lifting and scooping on the cheek.
2 Repeat for at least 30 seconds.

97

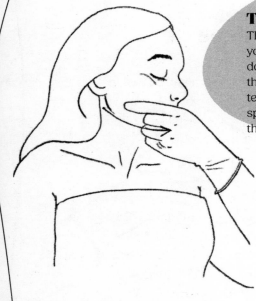

Top tip
This can feel a little sore, so if you do feel a tense spot, slow down and work directly on the area, gradually releasing tension. You may need to spend more time on one side than the other.

Jaw focus, 1-and-3

This move is particularly helpful for clients suffering with TMD.

1 From the set-up position, make sure the thumb located inside the mouth is all the way along the gum line, pressing back until it reaches resistance.
2 Starting on the masseter next to the ear, using the 1-and-3 technique (see p. 105), begin sculpting in, towards the centre of the face, moving very gradually, as you want to feel for the tension and begin to iron it out to release.
3 Repeat for at least 30 seconds.

Nasolabial focus – 1-and-3 technique

Accessing the muscle from both angles here makes this an incredible technique to help relax the tissues and muscles that connect into the nasolabial folds (creases to which the muscles of the cheek and those next to the nose and around the mouth connect).

1 Using your opposite hand, with your fingers on the outside of the face, move your thumb inside the mouth to sit underneath the nasolabial fold, then knead your fingers downwards towards the mouth. Your thumb should remain still and keep the pressure stable.

2 Now with the same 1-and-3 technique (see p. 105), sculpt the nasolabial fold, starting at the top of the fold next to the nostril, gradually buffing your way down to the corner of the mouth.

3 Repeat for at least 30 seconds.

Repeat all of the above on the opposite side. But first, take a look in the mirror and congratulate yourself. You'll notice less fluid retention, improved definition to the mid-face and more of a lift to the whole area.

NOSE

Clients frequently ask me whether facial massage can help with slimming the nose.

Our noses are predominantly made up of cartilage, and while we can absolutely sculpt muscles with exercise and techniques, this is less possible with cartilage. So the short answer to the question above is no, we cannot. However, the techniques here can help to relieve sinus pressure and built-up fluid around the nose which, in turn, helps to define its appearance. This, for many clients, can increase confidence, not to mention making them more comfortable.

Release and drain

This exercise hits the full sinus area, helping to release built-up fluid. Use it during the day, whenever you need that extra boost and release.

1 Begin by working on the sinus area, placing both index and middle fingers next to the nostrils (not directly on the nose itself).
2 Start with small, static, circular presses, upwards and outwards, with light to medium pressure, working just on the sinus area itself, next to the nostrils.
3 Work for up to 10 seconds.

Top tip
As you slide up to the brow, on the bridge
of the nose, be sure not to use firm
pressure – remember, the nose is cartilage
and light pressure is all that's needed.

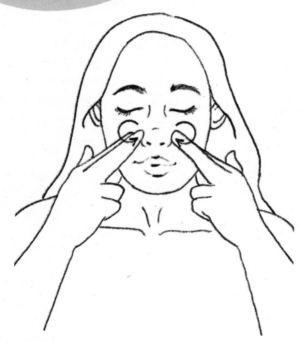

4 Now, with the same pressure, begin moving up, along
the sides of the nose, sliding onto the eyebrows,
stopping at the middle, before sliding back down again.

5 Repeat the sliding half-C move up and down with light
to medium pressure, for 30 seconds.

NASOLABIAL FOLDS

Being the place to which several facial muscles connect, it's no wonder this area gets a lot of use (and therefore raises a lot of concerns) – it's the hub of so many of our expressions.

Certain factors can cause these lines to deepen and look more prominent, such as smoking and sun exposure. But they are also known as smile or laughter lines and are a natural part of ageing. The techniques below will help to improve their appearance, softening but never removing them entirely. They are a natural fold of the anatomy and, as such, they are beautiful.

The techniques below are for daily use, as we know stress can unfortunately occur in day-to-day life, causing us to tense our muscles constantly. Therefore, the key tension-release moves are to be performed consistently for optimal results. I like to do the full sequence on one side at a time. However, I will detail all the options.

Vibrations

The full-face vibration technique from the 'Energise' section of your core routine *is* one to bring back here (see p. 71). If this is an area of focus for you, spend extra time on it when doing this move in that section. It's beneficial for lifting the tissue, enhancing blood flow to the area and preparing it for the moves you're about to perform.

Relax and release

Here, you're going to relax the muscles that activate the deep expression of the fold. This move can be done on both sides together or one side at a time for specific focus. And there's no need to rush it – it's a small move with the goal of deep relaxation.

1 Using your index and middle fingers, place the finger pads below the inner corner of the eye next to the nose (be sure not to place them on the nose bone itself). To get a better sense of where to place the fingers initially, raise your upper lip, as though in a snarling action – if you're in the correct position, you will feel your fingers lift with the muscle.

2 Apply medium pressure and begin small, localised, circular motions upwards and outwards, to relax the muscle. Sliding motions up and down are also great.

3 Gradually move downwards, along the nasolabial fold, stopping at the corner of the mouth and working back up.

4 Repeat up to 8 times.

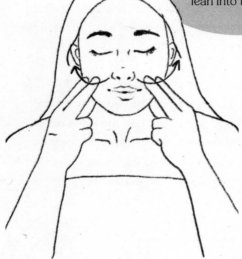

Top tip
Begin with slightly lighter pressure next to the nose and, as you glide underneath the cheekbone, you can begin to lean into the pressure.

Nasolabial sweeps

This move flows beautifully after the relax-and-release technique.

1 Using the same finger placement as above, begin at the same point, next to the nose and, with medium pressure, slide down the fold and outwards, along and underneath the cheekbone, finishing at the ear.

2 Repeat up to 8 times.

The 1-and-3 technique

A definite favourite, this can be done one side at a time for a specific focus or with two hands at once. (My preference is one side at a time, as you are then also able to support the surrounding tissue with the opposite hand.) This move helps to iron out the connective tissue, releasing blockages and promoting a smoothed appearance.

1 Starting on one side, use the hand of the side you're working on and place your four finger pads on to the nasolabial fold.

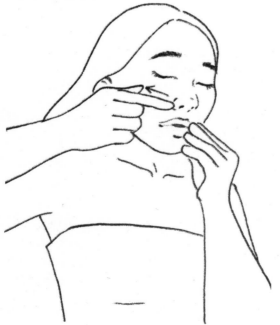

2 Place the length of your fingers of the opposite hand on the mouth with light to medium pressure (this creates tension and support, keeping the area taut). Be sure not to press so firmly that you create tension to the fold on the opposite side.

3 Now begin to move and slide outwards over the fold with the index finger first (1), and then as this finger pulls back use the other three together (3) to repeat the sliding motion outwards (1, 3, 1, 3 ...). Stay positioned just on the fold, not sliding out over the cheek – this is a localised move.

4 Repeat the move up and down the fold up to 8 times on each side, being mindful to slide outwards, not down.

Top tip

When performing this move it helps to lift your elbows out at a 90 degree angle, following the direction of the sculpt.

Nasolabial-fold rolling

This move takes some practice, but once you feel it and see the results, you'll love it! The technique is very similar to the neck rolling exercise on page 82.

1 Make sure there isn't so much product on the face that you can't grip the tissues.
2 Working one side at a time, using your index and middle fingers, as well as your thumb, pick up the tissue on the fold next to the corner of the mouth. Make sure you grab, pick up, pinch and lift the full tissue.
3 Allow your fingers to walk ahead of your thumb, gathering new skin as the thumb glides up the fold to be level with your nose. When you reach the top, lift off and start at the bottom again.
4 Repeat up to 8 times, then switch sides.

Top tip
Once mastered, this technique can be used across the face. I particularly like to perform it on the cheeks, as well as the lines around the neck.

Sweep and lift

This is a good move to finish off the sequence, to lift the tissues and drain away any remaining fluid.

1   Using the palm of one hand (still working one side at a time), separate the index and middle fingers and wrap the mouth with your index finger above the top lip and middle finger below the bottom.

2   Mould the hand into the cheek and sweep upwards and outwards with medium pressure, towards the ear.

3   Follow with the opposite hand, fingers pointing upwards, sweeping from the corner of the mouth, keeping the tissues lifted in one continuous move.

4   Repeat up to 8 times and finish with light pressure drains to the side of the neck before switching to the opposite side.

Top tip
The repetitive motion here keeps the tissues lifted – focus on making it one move, with the hands working one after the other.

EARS

Yes, we're talking ears – a place that often gets missed out entirely, so let's start by understanding why it's beneficial to turn your focus towards massaging this area.

Your ears are located in a very vascularised part of the face – an area with many lymph nodes – and therefore the place we work towards for drainage in many techniques. However, it is also full of nerves and home to many powerful acupressure points, creating sensations that resonate throughout the entire body. In Ayurvedic medicine, the ears are energy points connected to your organs and the entire body, meaning that ear massage can help to treat stress, as well as aches and pains in the body. It can also release endorphins and enhance the immune system.

Begin by removing all jewellery from the ear to allow full range of movement across the area.

Ear Vs

This is a move that appeared in the core routine (see p. 66 for your ear V pumping technique), but is a great one to spend more time on to see fantastic results. It works to stimulate the lymph nodes located around the ear.

Circular press and rotate

• •

1 Use the hand of the side you're working on and place the opposite hand in front of the ear, keeping the skin slightly taut.

2 Begin on the ear lobe itself, massaging in circular downward motions, using your index finger and thumb with medium pressure.

3 With each rotation, gradually work your way up the ear, along the edge of the cartilage and even more inside, covering the full ear.

4 Repeat up to 3 times.

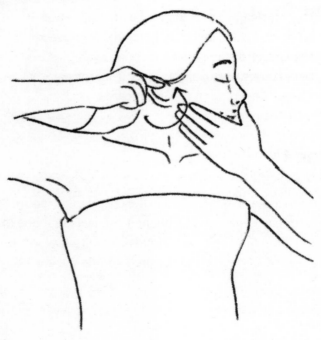

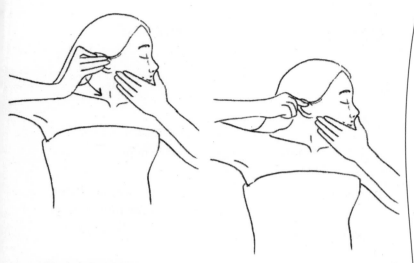

Ear focus – 1-and-3

Referring back to the 1-and-3 technique on p. 105, this is my main movement over this area.

1 Place one hand with your fingers over the ear horizontally and the other hand on your face near your ear, for support.
2 Massaging first with the index finger, then with the next three fingers together (the 1-and-3 method), begin sliding over the ear (massaging the ear itself) and the lymph nodes. This should create a light tugging sensation.
3 You should massage each part of the ear, from the top to the lobe.
4 Repeat on the other side once this side is done.

CHEEKS

This area can be prone to holding tension, and regular massage is invaluable in helping to combat this.

Core routine face squats

We're bringing back the face squats from the 'Stimulate' section of your core routine here (see p. 68). If this is your area of focus, be sure to spend the allocated time on this one.

Cheek hug and scoop

1 Adopting a prayer-like position with your hands, place your fingertips together in the centre of your forehead, with your thumbs next to the nose.
2 Sweep the base of your thumbs underneath the cheekbones, hooking as you glide along towards the ears, index fingers placed on the forehead for support. I find the thumbs work really well here for controlled pressure.
3 It's beneficial to repeat this move at least 8 times.

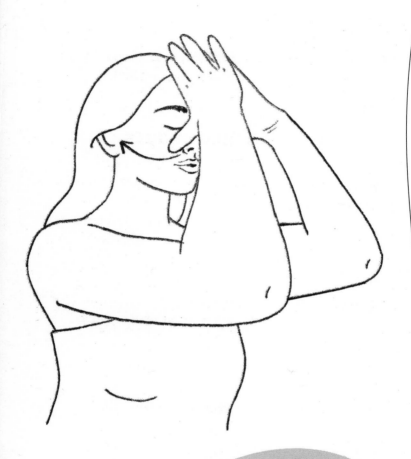

Top tip

Don't rush this move – if you feel tension, slow it right down and enjoy the release. Feels good, right?

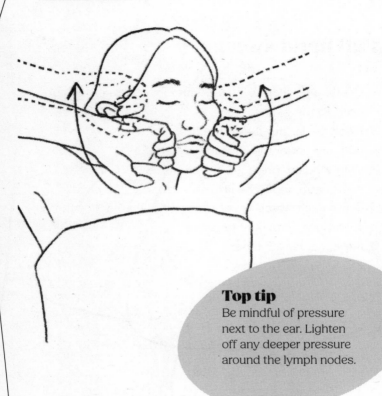

Top tip
Be mindful of pressure next to the ear. Lighten off any deeper pressure around the lymph nodes.

Knuckle hug and scoop

· ·

1 Lift your elbows out and place the flats of the knuckles next to your mouth, under your cheekbones, palms facing outwards.
2 With medium pressure, sculpt outwards to the ear, gradually. Don't rush through the move; slow down and feel for any tension.
3 It's beneficial to repeat this move at least 8 times.

Full hand sweeps

1 Create an L shape with the thumb and index finger on both hands.
2 Hook the Ls into the centre of the face with the thumb hugging under the chin and jawline.
3 With medium pressure, sweep out towards the ears, contouring under the jawline and across the cheeks.
4 Finish each sweep with a drain down the neck to the collarbone, with light pressure.
5 Repeat at least 3 times.

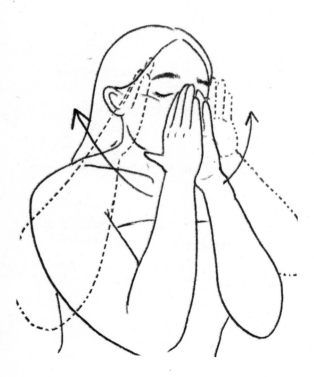

UPPER FACE

With no sebaceous activity, meaning no oil production like other parts of the skin, the eye area welcomes all the TLC.

Eye enhance

The eye movement in the upper-face lift in your core routine is a great place to start when beginning to target the delicate eye area (see p. 73).

Eye resistance

You're strengthening the muscles of the eye here, predominantly the orbicularis oculi (see p. 24).

1 Place the palms of your hands on your forehead with the little fingers covering the eyebrows.
2 Apply slight pressure with the little fingers, slightly lifting the eyebrow, but not enough to cause tension in the skin of the forehead.
3 Ensuring your shoulders are relaxed and posture upright and comfortable, begin to close your eyes and use your little fingers and hands as resistance, not allowing the eyes to close fully. This is resistance training to help strengthen the muscles.

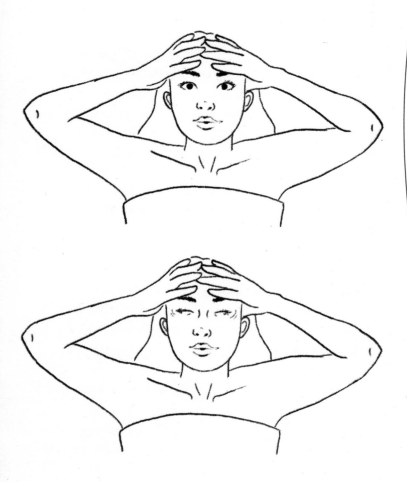

4 Try to close and resist for up to 3 seconds, then relax; do 20 repetitions.

Eye pump and glide

This massage technique focuses on drainage, with small pumps to continue the movement of fluid. Clients complain of puffiness in this area over any other, and that is down to the skin here being much thinner, meaning that any fluid build-up is more prominent.

This is my favourite move to encourage drainage, kick-start a flush to the area and brighten the eyes.

1 Using the middle and ring fingers on both hands, start next to the nose with small pumping motions, in a wave of light pressure from one fingertip to the other – a bit like a caterpillar. I like to spend a few seconds on the first spot next to the nose to kick-start the movement, before gliding gradually outwards with each wave and pump, until reaching the ears.

2 Repeat up to 8 times.

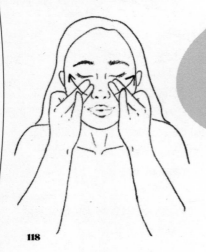

Top tip

Remember, you need light pressure here. The lymphatic system is relatively superficial, so light pumping motions are your best friend when it comes to encouraging drainage. You can repeat this type of technique over all areas of the face, following underneath the brow if your eyelids tend to get particularly puffy.

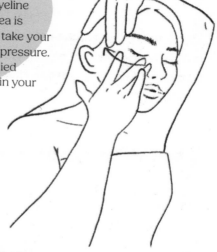

Top tip
You can work up to the eyeline here. As you know, the area is delicate and sensitive, so take your time and avoid too much pressure. These moves can be applied with eye cream as a step in your skincare routine.

Scoop and follow

This helps to brighten the under-eye area, stimulate blood flow and depuff.

1 Focusing on one eye at a time here, start with the right side. Using the ring and middle fingers of your right hand, sweep from the centre of the under-eye space, next to the nose, out and upwards to the top of the temple with light to medium pressure.

2 With the opposite hand, follow immediately after with the same fingers, sweeping up to the temple. This move works in a hand-after-hand motion, so that the lift is continuous.

3 Repeat up to 8 times with each eye individually.

Brow enhance

● ●

I recommend the same technique for the brow as you
did earlier for the eyes in your core routine (see p. 73),
as it helps to strengthen the muscles surrounding the
eye area.

Thumb press and lift

● ●

This is amazing for releasing tension in the upper face.

1 Adopting a prayer-like position with your hands,
place the base of the thumbs at the inner ends of
your two eyebrows, with your index fingers resting on
the forehead.
2 Start by spending some time on the inner part of the
eyebrows. With medium pressure, press your thumbs
in and slightly upwards for a few seconds on the
pressure points to release any built-up tension.
3 With both thumbs and still with medium pressure,
begin to slide through the eyebrows, slowly lifting
them as you glide.
4 Finish with the base of your thumbs on the temples
for a press and release.
5 Repeat up to 8 times.

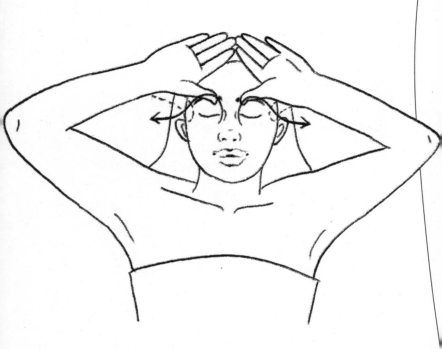

Top tip

For those who work at a computer screen or suffer with tension headaches, repeating this a few times throughout the day can help symptoms.

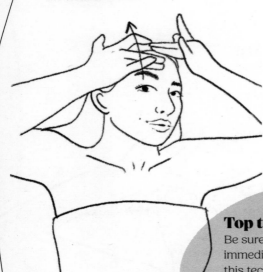

Top tip
Be sure to have a look at the immediate lift after performing this technique on one eyebrow. This is the initial result, and, with consistency and time, it will become long-lasting.

Full finger press and slide

1 Using a continuous motion, and on one eye at a time, place the length of the two fingers along one eyebrow (I like to use my middle and ring fingers for controlled pressure).

2 With medium pressure, slide up towards the hairline, immediately following with the other hand. Start this movement at the inner point of the eyebrow and work across, moving further out with each slide, until you're at the temple.

3 Repeat up to 8 times with both hands, one eyebrow at a time.

Two-finger hook

Once both sides have been worked on individually in the 'Full finger press and slide', try this technique on both together to stretch out and sculpt the area.

1 Create a hook-like shape with your index fingers and hook the inner sides into the head of the eyebrows, thumbs resting lightly on either side of the head for stability and support.

2 Apply light to medium pressure and slide up and through the eyebrows, creating a lift.

3 Finish at the middle of the eyebrows, keeping it specific to the between-the-eyebrow area.

4 Repeat up to 8 times.

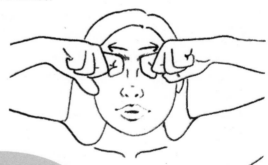

Top tip

If you wear glasses, or even suffer with eye strain, this is a great move for you, helping to relieve tension when the eyes feel heavy.

123

FOREHEAD

This area shows a lot of expression and emotion, which can contribute to fine lines and wrinkles on the skin. The techniques that follow are ideal for helping to improve the texture in this area.

Forehead resistance

This is a great move to strengthen the forehead, reducing the number of contractions to the connective tissue, in turn helping to iron out fine lines.

1 Place the palms of your hands on your forehead with the little fingers placed just above the eyebrows.
2 Apply very light pressure with all fingers but not enough to cause tension in the skin of the forehead, or so much that it affects your posture moving your neck forwards. This should feel comfortable.
3 Now attempt to lift your eyebrows, pulling a surprised expression. Your hands are there to resist the contraction and wrinkle formation of the frontalis and corrugator muscles.
4 Hold each contraction for 3 seconds.
5 Repeat 20 times.

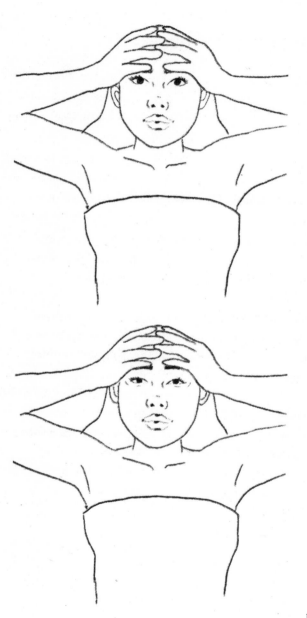

Muscle mobility

This is all about relaxing the key muscles of the eyes and forehead, as we know they work together with every movement. As mentioned previously, providing the muscles with deeper relaxation helps to further sculpt and lift – because if a muscle is stiff and tense, the techniques will not work as effectively. This move may seem strange to begin with, but you will notice immediately that the area feels lighter and lifted due to the relaxation and release in tension.

1 Lift your arm so your hand comes up and over your head, with the pads of all four fingers placed over the full length of the eyebrow.
2 Using medium pressure, begin to rotate the muscles with full circular motions in one direction using all four finger pads.
3 With every rotation slide upwards slightly towards the hairline, focusing more on the upward-lifting circular motions here, and giving minimal attention and pressure to the downward motion.
4 Repeat up to 8 times. Repeat on the opposite side with the opposite arm and hand.

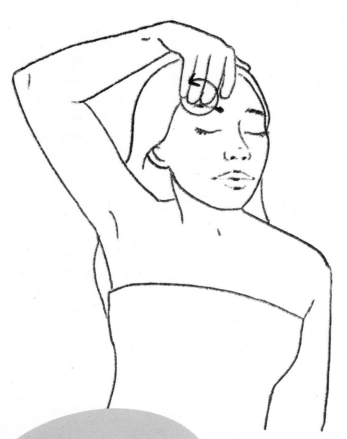

Top tip

Make sure your posture stays correct and comfortable throughout, shoulders down with your neck and back straight and head upright, not tilted. If you can (and you don't mind potentially getting product in the hair), continue into the hairline, finishing at the crown, as the muscle continues through to this point and it feels incredible!

Energise and plump

Following on from the 'Energise' practice in your core routine (see p. 74), this technique continues to build energy, blood and oxygen through the tissues, and is another one of my personal favourites. I'm going to give you two separate ways to perform the technique – you can choose the one that works best for you.

1 Be sure you have product for slip on the skin.
  With your dominant hand, all four fingers together and straight, place the length of your index finger on the forehead.
2 Keeping the fingers strong and straight, begin to buff from side to side with medium pressure, picking up the pace, building heat and friction.
3 Move along the full forehead gradually, working across the entire area.
4 You can then turn your fingers downwards and repeat the move, working up and down, covering every angle.
5 Repeat for up to 30 seconds.
6 The variation of this move uses the knuckle of your index finger to create a hook and buff with the knuckle. This provides more of a localised area of heat, which is great for targeting a small area or an individual fine line to plump.

Top tip
If this is an area you would like to focus on, add this technique into the 'Energise' section of your core routine for ease.

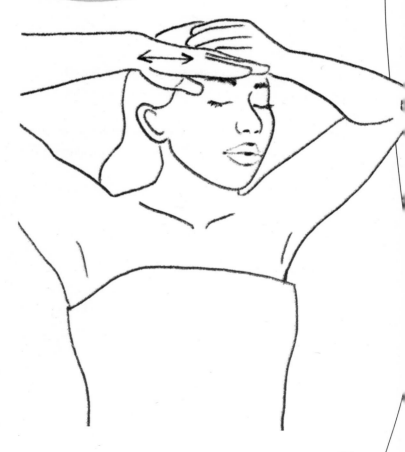

BETWEEN-THE-EYEBROWS FOCUS – THE 11s

For this area, it can be a good idea to work on the forehead first. The muscles work very closely together, especially here, so the techniques flow and enhance one another.

Frown resistance

This is a really great exercise to strengthen the small but mighty procerus muscle between the eyebrows.

1 Using the lengths of your middle and index fingers, place them along both eyebrows, leaving space on the procerus muscle.
2 Apply very slight pressure to both eyebrows and begin to attempt a frown, resisting with your fingers to prevent wrinkle formation.
3 Hold for 3 seconds.
4 Repeat 20 times.

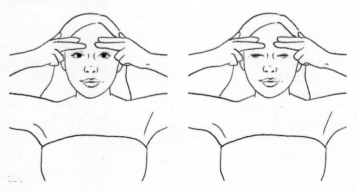

Energise and plump

A key move used in the previous forehead section (see p. 128), the energise-and-plump technique is extremely beneficial when working over fine lines and can be adopted all over the face. If between the eyebrows is a focus for you, repeat the move over this small area, using the lengths of your straight fingers. Work over the area for up to 30 seconds

Top tip

If you're very tense in this area, apply pressure to the point at the head of the eyebrow with a finger tip, and wiggle it slightly. This is a very small move that helps release blockages. Think of it as brushing someone's hair and using a gentle wiggle to help release a tangle.

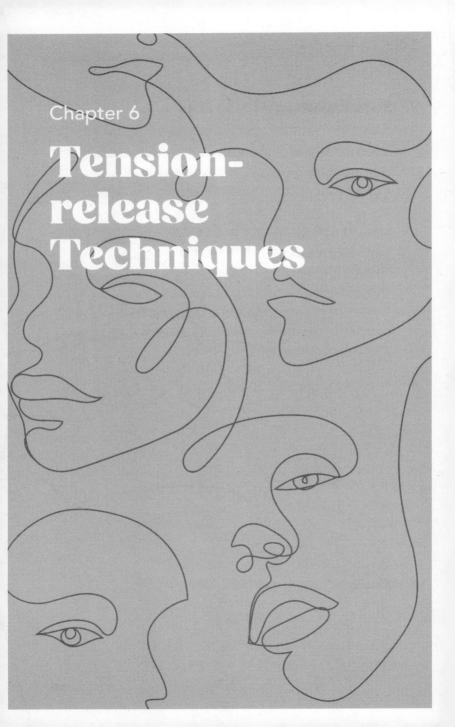

Chapter 6

Tension-release Techniques

So far, we've highlighted many of the visual benefits, but this section goes further, into the internal advantages. One thing in particular that facial massage is known to help with: tension release.

Some of the techniques we've already looked at can help with tension; however, the following are targeted more towards areas that commonly hold stress, with the aim of releasing any discomfort.

Be sure to take some time to rest and drink plenty of water after performing the practices in this chapter, as they can be intense.

Upper-body posture check

· ·

As I've said already, posture correction is important.
So firstly, check in with yourself. How are you sitting
right now? Is your upper body slightly hunched over?
If so, this one is definitely for you.

1 Begin by drawing your shoulders back and straight,
making sure they're not hunched forwards.
2 Drawing your attention to the neck, imagine you
have a string going through your head, keeping your
posture in line.
3 Focus on tucking the chin in, being mindful not
to draw it down, just straight back to line up with
the spine. It's easy to bring the shoulder forwards
while doing so, so make sure both are straight back
together. You'll feel a stretch and release at the
back of the neck.
4 Repeat up to 8 times.

Top tip
It's beneficial to almost
programme yourself to check in
and repeat this throughout the
day, realigning your stance, as
poor posture can contribute to
pain and discomfort.

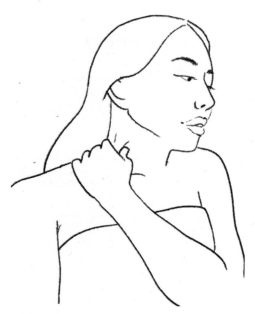

Neck release

This technique focuses on the sternocleidomastoid (SCM) muscles (see p. 25) on the sides of the neck. They run from the collarbone all the way up behind the ears. If you suffer with tension headaches and notice throughout the day that your shoulders creep up towards your ears, this can help. It takes a bit of practice, but the higher up you work, the more the release is usually felt.

1 Begin with one hand working on the opposite side of the face. I will use the left hand working on the SCM muscle of the right side.

2 Turn your head slightly to the right, looking in a diagonal direction (this makes it easier to grab the muscle). Gently pick up the SCM muscle at the base by the collarbone with your thumb and finger pads. It may take a few tries but once you've picked up and gripped the muscle – just light to medium pressure, not too firm – slowly turn your head to face the left in a diagonal position again, keeping hold of the muscle (if you turn too far, you will lose the grip).

3 Repeat this technique, each time working a little higher up the SCM muscle. You will feel a release and, potentially, pain in the back of the head – this would indicate you've found a trigger point, a hyper-irritable spot in the skeletal muscle that can be the cause of tension headaches.

4 Repeat a few times throughout the day if needed.

Top tip
Ease into this technique and don't apply too much pressure. When you get used to it, very slight wiggles around tense areas can be performed to release and ease.

Occipital press and hold

The point you are working with here is found on either side of your neck, at the base of your skull, directly above the shoulders. It's an incredible acupressure point, often referred to as heaven's pillar, and holding it helps to release an incredible amount of tension in the upper body. It is also known to provide emotional release.

1 Cradle the back of the head in your hands, placing your thumbs at the base of the skull.
2 Inhale deeply and on the exhale, press the length of your thumbs in and slightly upwards with light to medium pressure. You may need to move around the area a little until you find the sweet spot.
3 Repeat up to 8 times.

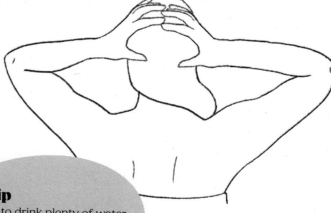

Top tip
Be sure to drink plenty of water and allow moments of rest as this point is incredibly powerful.

Hairline press and release

This helps to release pressure in the head and can ease pain from headaches.

1 Using all four finger pads on both hands, place them around the backs of the ears, at your hairline.
2 Lightly press with all four fingers in a line and rotate in small circular motions.
3 With each rotation, slowly move along the curve of the hairline, until you are at the top of the head.
4 Repeat up to 8 times.

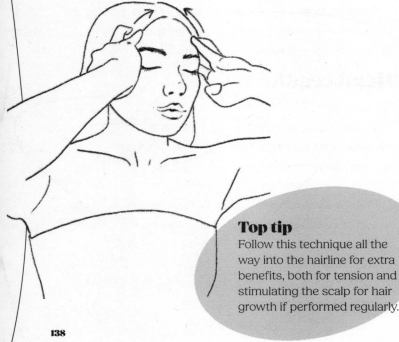

Top tip
Follow this technique all the way into the hairline for extra benefits, both for tension and stimulating the scalp for hair growth if performed regularly.

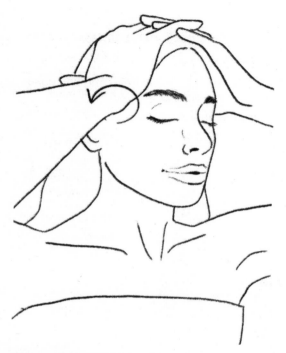

Head cradle

• •

This move is wonderful for releasing pressure – a pressure that can also refer up to the head and surrounding muscles.

1 Interlace your fingers together slightly, and cradle the top of your head, placing your palms on your temples. The top of your mandible (the jawbone) sits in this area; if you're unsure as to whether you're on the correct place, very gently grit your teeth and you will be able to feel the muscles bulge.

2 Make sure you're sitting comfortably and your posture is correct (shoulders down and neck straight), then, with your palms, apply medium pressure to the temples, moving them in circular motions up and outwards, giving the area a deep, releasing massage.

3 Repeat these circular motions on the same area up to 8 times.

4 Begin to rotate and glide backwards a little each time into the hairline, creating a release throughout the entire head.

Top tip

If you're particularly tense, this can feel a little uncomfortable, so as always, be extremely mindful of pressure – it should never hurt – and work with intention. These moves can be repeated a few times throughout the day when needed.

Brow squeeze

As the name suggests, this technique solely focuses on the eyebrows – one of the areas we most commonly hold stress and tension in.

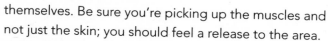

1   Starting in the middle of the eyebrows, using your thumbs and middle fingers, or index if you prefer, lift underneath the brows with your thumbs, and press with your fingers, squeezing the muscles themselves. Be sure you're picking up the muscles and not just the skin; you should feel a release to the area.

2   Continue along the length of the eyebrows, moving along slightly each time, until you are no longer able to lift the muscle.

3   Hold each point for up to 5 seconds and repeat up to 8 times.

Top tip
Pay attention to the thumb pressure here more than the fingers, as you don't want to press down on the eyebrows too much. The technique is about lifting the eyebrows upwards, also opening the eyes in the process.

141

Brow pressure spots

I like to work one side at a time here as this move hits the pressure points located through the eyebrows, so if you are feeling one side in particular, spend some time there to generate some comfort, and destress. This move can be performed without product, but if necessary, you can apply a drop to allow for slip, but be careful not to add too much.

1 Create a hook with your index finger and place your knuckle on the inner corner of your eyebrow with the opposite hand resting near by on the forehead for support, keeping the skin slightly taut.
2 Begin to glide through the eyebrow with light to medium pressure, slowly lifting it slightly upwards.
3 Pause and press as you gradually move along the eyebrow, holding each point up to 5 seconds, focusing on any area that feels particularly tense and finishing at the temple.

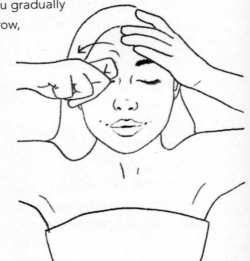

4 Repeat 3 times on each eye, tailoring where needed.

TMJs

Tension in the jaw is very common, the main culprit being the TMJs (temporomandibular joints). These are located in front of the ears, connecting the lower jaw to the skull, acting like a sliding hinge, to allow your jaw to open and close (with the assistance of several muscles, as well as ligaments). When these structures are not aligned, discomfort can occur with movement, leading to TMD (temporomandibular disorder), which presents as clicking or crunching noises in the jaw and pain that radiates down the neck and into the ears, as well as locking of the jaw and restricted mouth movement.

Many people experience this from time to time, one of the main causes being clenching or grinding the teeth (often due to stress), either during the day or at night. I've woken up many a morning with a tight jaw and know I've been clenching at night. Pain relievers, mouth guards and diet changes are commonly recommended to help with the discomfort, while massage is very popular and provides incredible relief. Of course, do visit your healthcare provider for advice if this is something you suffer with.

Here are some of my favourite at-home massage techniques specifically aimed at releasing built-up tension in the TMJ area, in turn easing discomfort. This area can be very tender, which is why these are light techniques that should never hurt – so be sure to go easy with your pressure and focus on your breath.

Hold and open

This move also highlights whether your jaw is opening slightly off centre, helping you to almost retrain the way you open and close your mouth.

1 Firstly, locate the TMJ on each side: using your middle fingers, slide in from the centre of your ears just a few centimetres, then slowly open your mouth and see if you can feel a slight bulge – that's your joint.
2 Place your fingers just over the joints and open your mouth very gradually while applying light pressure. Be sure to open very slowly, with your jaw opening straight and in line.
3 Hold for a few seconds when your mouth is fully open before releasing.
4 Repeat 3 times.

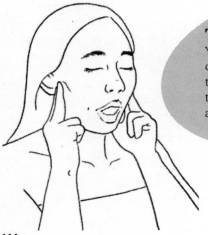

Top tip
You can also apply slight circular motions around the joint while performing this technique to help ease any tension.

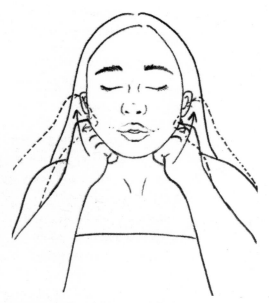

Knuckle release

This technique requires the addition of your chosen product for a slight slip and glide, but not so much that you're unable to grip the muscle. A favourite facial oil is great for this.

1 Apply the knuckles of both hands to the jawline, just above the bone on the lowest part of the masseter muscle (see p. 24).

2 With light to medium pressure (always check in with yourself to gauge this), slightly wiggle your knuckles side to side. The key thing to remember here is you're

not sliding on skin, you're applying pressure and simply rocking the muscle side to side very slightly – you'll absolutely feel it when you're in the correct place.

3 Spend a few seconds on each area before working your way up the masseter muscle very slightly each time, until you reach the TMJs, under the bone.

4 Repeat 3 times.

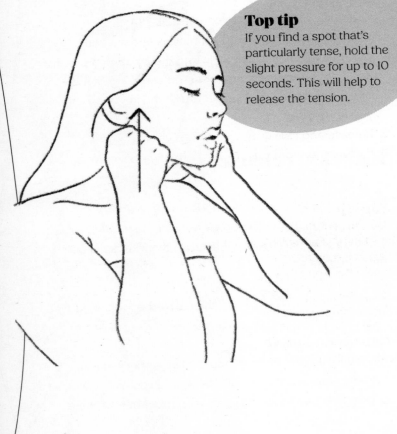

Top tip
If you find a spot that's particularly tense, hold the slight pressure for up to 10 seconds. This will help to release the tension.

Press and release

This is another of my favourite techniques – I always feel an immediate release when I do it. But I only use it if I'm feeling really tense and locked in my jaw.

1 Again, it's all about finding the correct spot here, which is underneath the corner of the jawbone, by the ear. Gradually press with light to medium pressure on both sides of the jawbone with your index fingers. You can perform very tiny circles to locate the area, then press and hold for up to 30 seconds. You can really feel this one – a dull ache radiating through the jaw itself while you're holding.

2 Release and slowly move the jaw.

3 Perform no more than twice, as this is a powerful one.

Top tip

You can perform this on one side at a time if you feel tension and discomfort more on one than the other. Focus on your breathing here.

Also, 'Jaw focus, 1-and-3' in the buccal massage section (see p. 98) is super beneficial for TMD. And it's a really nice way to finish off this sequence.

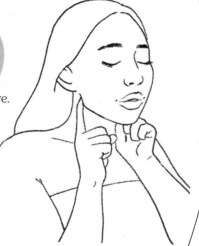

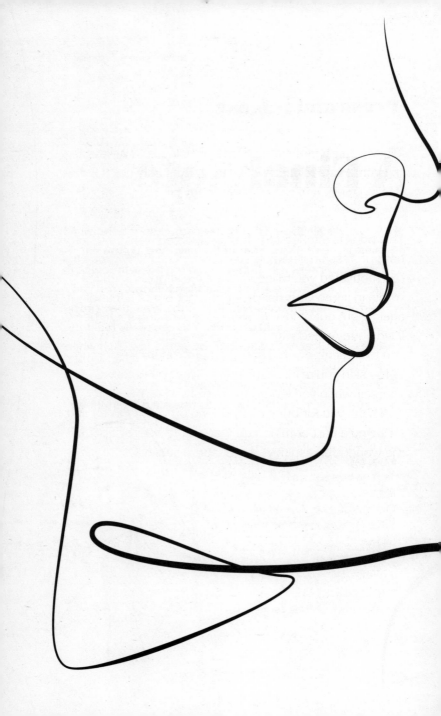

A Final Note

This book is a reflection of all I've learned from years of both professional and personal experience and I hope it has motivated you to incorporate the simple practices within in it into your daily routine – not out of a fear of ageing, but out of love for your face, working from the inside out. Armed with non-invasive techniques, I want you to feel empowered and, ultimately, incredibly proud of the skin you're in, changing the way you perceive yourself when you look in the mirror.

Thank you for bringing me along on your journey and for being a part of mine. I cannot wait to hear all about the wonderful results you're about to achieve.

Resources

For busting stress with guided mediations and breathing exercises

Headspace: Mindful Meditation app

Wim Hof Method: Breathing&Cold app

For the diet

The Candida Free Cookbook: 125 Recipes to Beat Candida and Live Yeast Free by Shasta Press (Callisto Media Inc. 2013)

For the results of studies in the benefits of facial massage

https://pubmed.ncbi.nlm.nih.gov/35416349/

https://onlinelibrary.wiley.com/doi/full/10.1111/srt.12345

For courses (coming soon)

www.sophieanneperry.com

Acknowledgements

Thank you to everyone who made this book possible, in particular the wonderful team at HarperCollins. Anna, it wouldn't have been possible without you and your talented mind.

My family, for always believing in me and being the most incredible support network a person could hope for. I love you more than words can say; you are my heroes.

J, for your love and support, I appreciate you more than you know.

Lade, my soul sister, for being by my side every step of the way.

To the best of friends – you know who you are! Thank you for always lending an ear and being my biggest fans, and for cheering me on after every word count milestone was reached; you're sensational.

To all the brands and industry professionals who have shared their wisdom with me over the past 14 years and kept my passion alive.

And finally, thanks to you all, my readers and supporters. To every single person who has attended a masterclass, picked up this book or shared themselves within this amazing community, I see you and thank you wholeheartedly.

About the author

Sophie Anne Perry is a beauty industry educator and practitioner living in London. With over 14 years in the beauty and wellness space, she is known for creating educational content, designing treatments and brand material, as well as hosting training, events and masterclasses for a global audience.

Her passion for all things wellness is the drive that has helped her build an ever-growing online community and a place to share knowledge that helps to change the conversation in beauty: to not focus on our flaws or concerns but to love the skin we're in. When she's not working, you're most likely to find Sophie trying new wellness innovations, fitness classes or exploring a new travel destination, drinking her favourite wine in the sunshine with loved ones.

@sophieanneperry_
www.sophieanneperry.com

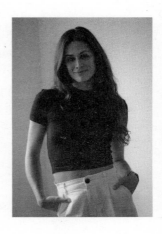